U0290292

[美国] 玛塔·L. 韦恩　[加拿大] 本杰明·M. 博尔克 著　彭诗意 译

传染病

牛津通识读本·

Infectious Disease

A Very Short Introduction

译林出版社

图书在版编目（CIP）数据

传染病 /（美）玛塔·L. 韦恩（Marta L. Wayne），（加）本杰明·M. 博尔克（Benjamin M. Bolker）著；彭诗意译.
—南京：译林出版社，2021.9
（牛津通识读本）
书名原文：Infectious Disease: A Very Short Introduction
ISBN 978-7-5447-8626-3

I.①传… II.①玛… ②本… ③彭… III.①传染病－防治 IV.①R51

中国版本图书馆 CIP 数据核字（2021）第 061635 号

Infectious Disease: A Very Short Introduction, *First Edition* by Marta L. Wayne and Benjamin M. Bolker
Copyright © Marta L.Wayne and Benjamin M. Bolker 2015
Infectious Disease: A Very Short Introduction, *First Edition* was originally published in English in 2015. This licensed edition is published by arrangement with Oxford University Press. Yilin Press, Ltd is solely responsible for this bilingual edition from the original work and Oxford University Press shall have no liability for any errors, omissions or inaccuracies or ambiguities in such bilingual edition or for any losses caused by reliance thereon.
Chinese and English edition copyright © 2021 by Yilin Press, Ltd
All rights reserved.

著作权合同登记号　图字：10-2020-86 号

传染病　[美国] 玛塔·L.韦恩　[加拿大] 本杰明·M.博尔克 / 著　彭诗意 / 译

责任编辑　陈　锐
装帧设计　景秋萍
校　　对　孙玉兰
责任印制　董　虎

原文出版　Oxford University Press, 2015
出版发行　译林出版社
地　　址　南京市湖南路 1 号 A 楼
邮　　箱　yilin@yilin.com
网　　址　www.yilin.com
市场热线　025-86633278
排　　版　南京展望文化发展有限公司
印　　刷　江苏扬中印刷有限公司
开　　本　635 毫米 ×889 毫米　1/16
印　　张　14.75
插　　页　4
版　　次　2021 年 9 月第 1 版
印　　次　2021 年 9 月第 1 次印刷
书　　号　ISBN 978-7-5447-8626-3
定　　价　39.00 元

版权所有 · 侵权必究

译林版图书若有印装错误可向出版社调换。质量热线：025-83658316

序　言

谢　青

人类浩荡的文明史进程始终离不开与传染病的斗争，从重溃古希腊文明的雅典大瘟疫到中世纪席卷整个欧洲的黑死病，再到20世纪80年代开始遍及全球并令人闻之色变的艾滋病，直至眼下肆虐全球且尚未平息的“黑天鹅事件”新型冠状病毒肺炎；人类一度对来势汹汹的“敌人”束手无策，好在医学的快速发展让我们由守转攻逐渐掌控了这场鏖战的主导权。溯因来看，传染病由各类细菌、真菌、病毒、衣原体、支原体、立克次体、寄生虫等病原微生物引起，侵袭人类的方式包括但不限于呼吸道传播、粪口传播和体液传播。毫不夸张地说，人类和病原微生物的关系并非此消彼长而是共同进化，博弈双方针对彼此的“阿喀琉斯之踵”不断更新进攻策略以瓦解对方的惯用战术，往复循环，直至停火期，并须时刻提防对方卷土重来。在这个漫长的交战过程中，双方的作战能力都较交战伊始上升了好几个维度。

以人类抗争细菌感染为例，抗生素这一“武器”在投用初期可谓立竿见影、直击命脉，有效而稳定地控制了一系列敏感菌对机体造成的损害。然而，在我们喜悦未久之际，细菌已悄然实行了“破壁”方案，耐药菌株发生菌种替换，特异性阻绝原先抗生素的作用位点，人类由此不得不开发更强劲的新型武器进行围剿。这又进一步刺激细菌予以“兵来将挡，水来土掩”的反击，经多次对垒之后，以MRSA为代表的“超级细菌”诞生了。野火烧不尽，春风吹又生，这种具多重耐药特性的“佼佼者”宣告了细菌应对人类治疗策略的胜利，而从某种程度上看，这也是人类绞尽脑汁应战却始料未及催生出的“副产品”。

人类社会消灭一切现有的病原微生物从而消灭传染病是不现实的，不过也不是没有成功的案例。得益于疫苗接种，天花成为第一个被人类消灭的传染病，这给予了我们在探索传染病管控方面极大的信心。人类对事物的恐惧往往来源于无知，大众对“流行病”“烈性传染病”等概念易存在诸如“触之即死”“不可治愈”等危言耸听的思维误区，而对疾病了解得愈深，我们便不再畏惧它，从而正视解决问题的方法。牛津通识读本《传染病》正是这样一本面向普罗大众的入门级科普读物，它深入浅出地解释了传染病学领域常用但晦涩的高壁垒术语而使其生动有趣，譬如“基本再生数R_0”“仓室模型”“抗原漂移”“Koch法则”等，以流感病毒、HIV、霍乱弧菌和疟原虫等严重危害人类健康的病原体为案例，娓娓道来各类传染病的特性，以及人类应对这些严峻挑战的成功经验与不足，使我们能更辩证地看待人类与病原体的共存。

毋庸置疑，传染病学研究的不断发展，也带动了微生物学、现代免疫学、预防医学和生态学研究的持续进步，但也正是基于人类对某些病原体的驾驭，在新型疗法和预防手段不断涌现的同时，与传染病相关的不良衍生事件也在人类近现代史上频发：首当其冲的就是第二次世界大战时期日本731部队密谋的细菌战和以2001年美国炭疽攻击事件为典型的生物恐怖主义袭击，而利用任何形式将病原体进行人为传播的兽行都应被强力谴责；其次，假借防范艾滋病的名义进行婴儿CCR5基因编辑非法操作的贺建奎事件，也给学界敲响了重大传染病防治不应违背伦理的警钟。此外，曾轰动一时的“伤寒玛丽”则让大众进一步意识到，无症状感染者这一类特殊感染群体的存在，已成为传染病防治时控制传染源中最易被忽略但也最为关键的一环，若掉以轻心未能及早发现，后果将不堪设想，并且还会加深大众心中对这一偏见性社会隐喻的芥蒂。

不难看出，传染病防治应纳入的考量，不只是就病原体和疾病本身而言，它更是一个公众问题，与人文、伦理、社会学彼此交融。我国自经历2003年的SARS、2009年的H1N1猪流感和2013年的H7N9禽流感等重大传染病事件以来，在传染病防治领域中所做出的巨大贡献国内外均有目共睹，新冠疫情下毅然决然的防控策略，更体现出我们在直面传染病时的大国担当和中国决心。这些不断累积的中国经验不仅是对传染病防治的最佳解读，也是在公众当中普及传染病学知识的最佳手段，只有不断增强公众对传染病的认知，才有可能在未来应对突发传染病的过程中不断取得胜利。

目　录

致 谢

献给查理、诺玛、塔拉并（纪念）詹戈。

我们感谢美国国立卫生研究院的部分支持。我们要感谢牛津大学出版社善解人意且专业的编辑人员，特别是凯茜·肯尼迪，以及提供了友好评论和技术性建议的同事：拉斯托姆·安提亚、亚尼斯·安东诺维奇、茱莉亚·巴克、罗宾·布什、乔纳森·杜绍夫、戴维·厄恩、戴维·希利斯、林塞·基根、马尔姆·基尔帕特里克、亚伦·金、马克·利普西奇、格伦·莫里斯、朱丽叶·普利安、马可·萨利米和戴维·史密斯。毋庸讳言，我们对任何剩余的错误或过度简单化负有全部责任。

第一章

引　言

我们常说"有感染力的歌词"和"病毒式的视频"。这些与传染病有关的比喻渗透在21世纪的西方流行文化中。人们对下一次传染病大流行的担忧，正在世界范围内悄然升温。传染病危机来来去去：在过去的十年里，生物恐怖主义、SARS、H1N1流感和埃博拉病毒轮番出现，令人忧心。

早在20世纪70年代，医生就大胆地宣布终结传染病的时代已经开始。他们认为，用于预防病毒的疫苗和治疗细菌感染的广谱抗生素可以应对任何传染病的威胁。但传染病从未消失，甚至从未得到缓解。就在医生宣布胜利之际，抗药性**金黄色葡萄球菌**（英国小报中报道的一种"食肉细菌"）正在医院中传播（日本在20世纪50年代曾经历过抗药性细菌的暴发，但当时西方国家很少注意到这些流行病）。20世纪80年代，随着HIV的出现，传染病的形势更为严峻，时至今日，HIV疫苗的研发仍举步维艰。在意识到传染病的新威胁后，美国医学研究所在20世纪90年代初提出了名词"新发与再发传染病"。　1

传染病是一种由病原体引起的，能在人与人或其他生物之间传播的疾病。相反，非传染性疾病，例如心脏病、糖尿病、阿尔茨海默病，则是由于环境和遗传基因的共同作用导致的。引起传染病的生物被称为**病原体**或**寄生虫**。虽然生物学家曾经只用“寄生虫”来描述相对较大的致病生物，如绦虫或蜱虫，但现在也包括了微生物（病毒、细菌和真菌），这使两个术语的含义几乎相近。

我们之所以害怕传染病，正是**因为**它具有传染性。肉眼通常无法看见传染病的病原体，故在很大程度上，接触病原体是不可避免的，除非完全不与人接触。1842年，埃德加·爱伦·坡在他的小说《红死魔的面具》中描述了人们对传染病的恐惧，并指出断绝人类之间的接触来避免传染病是无效的。在该书中，一群贵族隐居到一个与世隔绝的地方，想躲避一场名为“红死病”的瘟疫。最终，一个盛装打扮的陌生人混进化装舞会，尽管采取了预防措施，但所有贵族都死于这种疾病。

不管爱伦·坡书中的贵族们所采取的避免疾病传播的措施多么不见成效，然而在人类历史的长河里，这一直是对抗传染病的唯一途径。直至19世纪中叶，疾病传播的机制才被世人所知，故在此之前，人类社会面对流行病所能做的就是切断与疫区的联系。1665年，为了躲避伦敦鼠疫，艾萨克·牛顿退居乡下，偶然之中，创立了微积分并发现了万有引力定律。同年，英国的埃姆村为防止鼠疫蔓延，自愿封村隔离，最终有一半以上的村民死亡。“隔离”一词现指强制隔开潜在感染者，以避免传染给他人，该词起源于“四十天”，即在威尼斯，为确保船上人员没有得瘟疫，船只必须在城外等待四十天。

隔离（至少好于坡书中的措施）确实能阻止传播，但从根本上来说，这是被动的，因为只有当人们意识到严重的疾病威胁时，才会采取隔离措施。这些措施只对未感染的健康人群有用，而对已感染者或不幸被困在隔离区的未感染者没有太大的意义。另一方面，只要我们对疾病的传播方式有所了解，隔离措施对任何疾病都是有效的（因为鼠疫是由鼠蚤传播的，所以只阻止人与人之间的接触但不灭鼠是无济于事的）。

隔离是为了保护群体而不是个体。随着医学水平的提高，公共卫生官员开始将工作重心从保护人群转移到保护个人。免疫接种是指，通过毒性温和的病原体菌株或毒素等外来物质刺激免疫系统从而保护人体的过程，是传染病个体防控工作中的第一个重大突破。18世纪初，天花免疫接种已在非洲、中国、印度和土耳其广泛开展。1721年，英国驻土耳其大使的妻子玛丽·沃特利·蒙塔古夫人将天花疫苗引入英国，引起了西方民众的关注，而更引人注目的是，同年由马萨诸塞州波士顿殖民城市的牧师科顿·马瑟推广的一项“实验”。面对天花的暴发，马瑟和他的医学同事扎布迪尔·博伊尔斯顿违背了大多数波士顿同胞的意愿，贸然推行免疫接种。尽管有几位患者死亡，但这一实验证实了一种物理隔离的有效替代方法：免疫接种能保护个体免受感染，并且不限制人们的自由活动。

马瑟和博伊尔斯顿的实验还说明了，为了个人利益而控制疾病和为了群体利益而控制疾病之间的伦理冲突。成功接种疫苗后的波士顿市民是安全的，但在接种后的几天里，他们可能会把疾病传染给没有保护措施的个人。大多数现代疫苗制剂所含的是非感染性物质，所以这一特殊的问题在今天已不那么令人担忧，但个人健康和公共健康之间的冲突仍然存在。

大多数免疫接种只能防止健康人被感染，但不能治愈感染者。20世纪中叶，随着抗生素的出现，个体水平的传染病防控又向前迈进了一步。抗生素最初是从常见的家庭霉菌和细菌中提取出来的，后来在实验室中合成，可以用来治疗感染患者。治愈传染病的可能性也减轻了人们对隔离的恐惧，在此之前，隔离被视为死刑。

在治疗有害细菌感染的抗生素和预防脊髓灰质炎、麻疹和百日咳等疾病的新型有效疫苗的浪潮之间，对于20世纪70年代的公共卫生官员来说，没有传染病的未来似乎已经触手可及。然而，他们很快就面临许多传染病无法通过个体层面措施得到有效控制的难题。疫苗是通过激活人体的免疫系统发挥作用的，因此，对于像疟疾或艾滋病等已经进化出逃避免疫系统策略的传染病病原体来说，疫苗的研发要困难得多。抗生素只对细菌有效，而对其他微生物，如病毒或真菌无效（虽然确实存在抗病毒和抗真菌的化学物质，但这些物质远不如抗生素作用范围广泛并且有效）。20世纪末，随着人们认识到传染病终究没有被征服，研究方向开始重新转向群体层面的控制。

到目前为止，我们将治疗方案根据主要是针对群体（隔离）还是个体（免疫/疫苗接种、抗生素）进行了划分。然而，进一步研究发现，抗生素和免疫接种既有助于保护群体，也能造福于接受治疗的患者。药物治疗可以减少传染病的影响，因为康复的人也不会传染他人。因此，治疗感染患者可以减少传播。疫苗预防感染是指一些潜在的传染性接触（感染者打喷嚏或性行为等活动，与传染病的传播途径有关）不会对已进行免疫接种的人造成威胁，从而再次减少了传播。这种所谓的**群体免疫**缩小了流行病的传播范围，甚至防控效果更优于接种疫苗所起到的直接作用。如果对足够多的人进行免疫接种，就可以充分减少传播，从而杜绝某种流行病的发生。若是能在全球范围内采取这样的措施，那么相应的疾病就会被消灭（就像天花一样，环保主义者并不担心它的灭绝）。

如果问题仅仅只是某些疾病较难控制，我们在防治传染病的斗争中仍然会取得进展，虽然比较缓慢。现代分子生物学为人类提供了很多种新型抗病毒药物，甚至连疟疾这样的疑难疾病的疫苗也在研制中。但人类和传染病病原体都是生物，所有的生物都经历着生态和进化的演变，这让传染病成为一个动态的目标。我们逐渐认识到人类（及瘟疫）与生命之轮息息相关，个体水平的防控措施未能让我们脱离出生命之轮，这推动了当今传染病研究的转变。

生态过程

尽管我们试图否认，但人类受制于生态学法则。我们掌控着我们环境的大部分。机动车取代大型捕食者，成为暴力性死亡的主要类别；我们消灭了大多数潜在的竞争对手，并且驯化了处于食物链下端的生物。但是，传染病仍然将我们与全球生命网络联系在一起。

5

最重要的疾病生态学联系是**人畜共患病**，即新发疾病由动物**宿主**传染给人类：埃博拉（病毒可能来源于蝙蝠）可能是最引人注目的例子，但很多我们尚未掌控的新发疾病都与动物相关：SARS、禽流感（H5N1）和汉坦病毒，这些都是较为人们熟知的例子。事实上，几乎所有的传染病都是动物源性疾病，而且大多数新发传染病都是人畜共患病。由于很难针对未知疾病进行疫苗接种或开展药物研发，所以这些新疾病威胁的出现令人恐惧：我们不知道何时会出现一种“超级传染病”。

人畜共患病并非新鲜事。天花被认为是至少在一万六千年前，由啮齿动物传播给人类的；麻疹是在9世纪左右，由牛传播给人类的；HIV则是在20世纪初通过猴子和黑猩猩传染给人类的。然而，无论是在热带雨林（HIV和埃博拉）还是在温带气候地区的郊区（莱姆病），人口的快速增长和土地利用的变化都增加了人类与动物的接触。

除了与动物有更密切的接触外，全球人口的流动速度也在加快。与17世纪艾萨克·牛顿逃离瘟疫，或19世纪爱伦·坡创作《红死魔的面具》时相比，人与人之间的接触导致疾病传播的速度更快，距离也更远。以前传播范围局限在有限区域（一般在发展中国家）的传染病现在可以迅速扩大其传播范围。不仅人类传染病是这样，影响其他物种的疾病也是如此，这些疾病的传染源由人类通过行李、旅行中所吃的食物或鞋子进行传播。人类的旅行和商贸活动可能通过运输动物（尤其是昆虫）**病媒**间接传播疾病，将疾病从某一生物体传染给另一生物体。例如，在国际二手轮胎贸易上，传播登革热的病媒伊蚊。除了病媒，人们有时也会转移人畜共患病的宿主。1989年，非洲以外地区的首位埃博拉病毒感染者，传染源是从菲律宾进口用于动物实验的猴子（食蟹猕猴）。幸运的是，所涉及的特殊菌株（埃博拉—雷斯顿型）对人类无害。

人口流动性的增加将病媒和宿主传播到新的地区，环境变化让它们能够在新家园中繁衍。随着全球气候变化，动物，特别是对温度敏感的昆虫，可能会入侵温带的新地区。虽然这个话题仍然存在争议，但许多气候学家和一些流行病学家相信，在区域气候变化的影响下，登革热和疟疾等蚊媒疾病已经在向新的人群中扩散。人类居住和经济活动模式导致的更为局部的环境变化，将会对传染病的传播产生更大的影响。例如，传播登革热的蚊子幼虫在如旧轮胎和家用水箱大小的水体中生长。一般来说，随着发展中国家人民从农村移居到日益繁荣的城市，他们将面临更严重的污水问题（传播霍乱和其他水媒疾病），并遇到了新的、不同种类的携带疾病的昆虫。

进化过程

生态学不断地让我们面临新的流行病，但进化让情况变得更严重：即使是我们有所了解的传染病，正当我们试图防控它们时，也会发生变化。作为为生存而战的生物，传染病并不是偶然逃脱我们的控制的。实际上，这是自然选择的结果。传染病在不断地变化，我们越努力与它对抗，它变化得越快。疾病生物学家经常引用刘易斯·卡罗尔所著《爱丽丝漫游奇境》中红桃皇后的话："你需要尽全力奔跑，才能保持在同一个地方。"

对于每一种疾病的预防策略，传染病都有相应的进化对策。细菌并非因人类使用抗生素而产生抗药性：科学家们在从三万年前的冻土中提取的DNA中，发现了类似于现代基因变体的抗生素抗药性基因。这并不奇怪，因为人类并没有发明抗生素。相反，抗生素是在真菌中发现或者产生的，真菌已进化出对抗细菌的策略。然而，抗生素在医药和农业中的广泛使用，使得对一种或多种抗生素产生抗药性的细菌能够战胜对抗生素敏感的细菌。其他生物，如引起疟疾的原生动物，也对治疗药物产生了抗药性。当艾滋病患者服用单一药物而不是应用联合多种药物的“鸡尾酒”疗法时，病毒在短短几周内就会在体内产生抗药性。病原体进化出对疫苗和药物的耐受性，但方式不尽相同。不是抗药性基因在病原体种群中传播，而是发生了**菌种替换**，即以前对疫苗有免疫力的罕见类型占据了整个菌群。

尽管与细菌和病毒相比，蚊子的数量较少，出生率也较低，因此进化速度要慢得多，但蚊子也找到了进化对策来应对我们的疾病控制策略。在发达国家，随着雷切尔·卡森等人敲响了滴滴涕对野生动物产生有害影响的警钟，滴滴涕被停用了，但即使在发展中国家，基于滴滴涕的病媒控制策略的效果也是短暂的，因为在大规模喷洒方案开始后的十年内，蚊子就已经进化出对滴滴涕的抗药性了。

8

传染病生物学的每一个方面都在不断演变，不仅仅是抵抗或规避控制措施的能力。生物学家已经注意到，一种疾病的毒性——对宿主的危害程度，是病原体进化的特征。通常情况下，毒力温和的传染病的病原体会发生突变，使它们的致病力更强。西尼罗河病毒出现于20世纪90年代末，这种病毒发生单一突变后，对乌鸦的致死性显著增强，但尚未明确这种突变是否也与西尼罗河病毒在人体中的毒力增强有关。

虽然突变是随机的，但自然选择的进化却并非如此：病原体一旦发生突变，其后续生物学行为的成败取决于生态条件。生物学家保罗·埃瓦尔德率先指出了病原体生态条件的变化，比如从人与人之间的直接传播转变为水媒传播，可能促使传染病致病力变得更强。全球航空旅行的兴起，可能会推动疾病的进化和生态变化：一些生物学家指出，空间上分散的种群之间的混合可能会增强病原体毒性。

展　望

考虑到这些挑战，消灭传染病——20世纪的动人之歌——似乎毫无希望，而仅仅依靠保护个体的防控策略似乎站不住脚。看来我们必须学会与传染病共存，而不是消灭它。然而，我们也必须努力减少传染病带来的痛苦。因此，21世纪以来，人们从试图消灭传染病的病原体，转变为试图了解、预测和管理传染病在群体层面的传播。在这种新的理论努力中，主要的工具不是神 9 奇子弹的技术，而是生态学和进化学科。生态学，因为理解生态关系有助于我们理解传播的周期。进化，因为病原体既会自行进化，也会随着我们的防控努力而进化。 10

第二章

不同规模的传播

传播定义了传染病。当一个人将疾病传给另一个人时，就会发生传播：严格来说，当一个宿主体内的病原体成功地进入另一个宿主体内并定居时，就会发生传播。

传播的方式多种多样。例如，在流行性感冒（一种呼吸系统疾病）的传播过程中，感染者肺细胞产生的病毒颗粒首先会通过咳嗽或打喷嚏进入周围的空气。这些感染性颗粒可以在空气中或自然环境中的表面短暂存活，因此只需要极少的接触就可以在人与人之间直接传播。接触者可以直接吸入病毒颗粒，或者可以通过触摸被飞沫污染过的物体表面沾染病毒。然后，这些病毒携带者会通过触摸自己的面部将病毒颗粒转移进鼻子；鼻子内空气的自然流动会将病毒吸入呼吸道。在呼吸道里，病毒颗粒会入侵易感细胞，并继续它们在宿主体内从一个细胞传播给另一个细胞的循环。

许多病毒，包括流感和引起腹泻的病毒，如轮状病毒，可以在自然环境中存活数日，聚积在被称为**污染物**的特定类型物体上。你是否注意到打领结的男医生突然增多了？这种时尚表现是对健康研究人员将标准领带鉴定为污染物的回应。流感病毒甚至可以在纸币上存活数天，特别是与“鼻咽分泌物”（鼻涕）混合时，但实际上我们并不知道这种传播途径在真正的流行病中是否重要。

病原体通常依赖于人与人之间的体液交换进行直接传播，而一旦离开人体温暖潮湿的环境，病原体的感染性颗粒几乎会瞬间死亡，例如HIV（见第四章）和淋病等性传播疾病。虽然在人类进化史的大部分时间里，性接触是最常见的体液交换形式，但这些病原体也可以通过输血或吸毒者共用注射器等更现代的体液交换方式传播。

其他无法在自然环境中生存的病原体已经进化到利用其他生物，特别是吸血昆虫和螨虫作为从一个宿主传播到另一个宿主的病媒。与直接在同一物种的两个宿主之间传播相比，这种传播策略需要更多的生物机理参与。在极端情况下，如疟疾等传染病的病原体，具有复杂的生命周期（见第六章），其在病媒蚊子体内经历了重大转变。事实上，从寄生于蚊子体内的疟原虫的角度来看，人类只是将它自己传播给另一只蚊子的一种便捷方式。

其他传染病的病原体在宿主体外会存活更长时间。像霍乱（见第五章）、伤寒和军团病等疾病的病原体可以在水中生存，可通过饮用水或空调系统进行传播。炭疽病——能迅速杀死宿主，降低直接在动物宿主间传播的可能性——的病原体炭疽杆菌产生的孢子，可在自然环境中持续存活数年，当动物摄取附着在土壤颗粒上的孢子时，就会被感染。许多真菌，如某些种类的

12

曲霉菌，主要为非寄生类生物，但也会在人类宿主体内繁殖，特别是宿主的免疫系统因压力或感染其他疾病而减弱时（这被称为**机会性**传染病，与大多数病原体的**专性**依赖相反。如果有宿主可得，机会性感染就可以在宿主体内生存，但不需要依赖宿主来完成它们的生命周期）。水陆两栖真菌**蛙壶菌**（见第七章）与非致病性土壤真菌密切相关，但据我们所知，它本身是一种专性寄生虫，只能在自然环境中存活数周。

相遇和相容筛选

根据克劳德·库姆斯的工作，我们可以将传染病传播过程分为三个阶段：（1）病原体从原宿主的身体内部转移到自然环境中；（2）通过自然环境，或者通过中间病媒或宿主的身体，病原体转移到接收宿主；（3）病原体从自然环境侵入接收宿主体的特定部位，如血液、肺或肝脏，并进行繁殖。这三个阶段共同构成了**相遇筛选**。

病原体进入新宿主的身体后，必须克服生理、生化和免疫方面的障碍后才能进行繁殖。换言之，即使病原体可以通过相遇筛选，但也必须与新宿主在生物学上相容；这一最后阶段被称为**相容筛选**。宿主可以通过抗病基因突变关闭其相容筛选，例如镰刀状细胞的血红蛋白基因能抗疟疾。只要宿主免疫系统正常，机会性真菌感染通常不会发生。然而，为了阻断大多数病毒性疾病，宿主的免疫系统需要在自然情况下或通过疫苗接种，提前与病原体相遇。

相遇和相容筛选必须都打开，病原体才能成功传播。公共卫生措施可以关闭相遇筛选，这在流行性传染病的早期阶段尤

13

为重要。虽然药物或疫苗可以关闭相容筛选，但并不是始终可用的。

关闭相遇筛选的方法包括简单的预防策略，如隔离（见第一章）。此外，还包括环境策略，如改善卫生设施，控制水媒疾病，或灭蚊虫、蜱虫，阻止虫媒疾病。另一类防控策略是说服民众改变自身行为。其中包括美国疾病控制和预防中心建议“捂嘴咳嗽”来防止流感，并且注意避免西尼罗河病毒等蚊媒疾病：傍晚时待在室内，穿长裤和长袖，并使用驱虫剂。虽然改变人们的行为方式很难，但这通常是控制疾病最经济的方法。不需要注射或服用可能有不良副作用的药物，行为方式的改变甚至可以预防未知病原体的侵入。即使已对目前所有已知的疾病进行了筛查，避免与陌生人有体液交换的行为仍然是预防传染病的一个良好举措。

流行病动力学

在个体层面上，很容易理解相遇和相容筛选：如果能防止自然环境中的感染性微粒侵入人体，或者如果通过免疫接种预防疾病的感染，就可以维护自身安全。我们需要数学模型了解这些筛选在群体层面的效果，例如，确定免疫接种或隔离是否能阻止流行病。在生物学家开始了解疾病传播的机制时，数学家们就开始研发模型，用以描述相遇和相容筛选在群体层面上的影响。早在1760年，瑞士著名数学家和科学家家族的成员丹尼尔·伯努利，就使用了一个数学模型来描述天花免疫接种（即关闭部分人的相容筛选）可以在多大程度上改善公共健康。伯努利的结论是，免疫接种可以将出生时的预期寿命增加10%，从大

14

约二十七岁增加到三十岁（由于婴儿和儿童死亡率高，18世纪人类出生时的预期寿命非常短）。

伯努利的模型只考虑了免疫接种的直接好处，而忽略了对群体免疫的关键见解。免疫接种保护已注射过疫苗的人，但也减少了疾病的流行，从而让未接种疫苗的人间接获益。要根除疾病，不需要完全关闭相容和相遇筛选（即人们100%接种疫苗，或全天候防止传播）；只需要充分减少传播，使每例传染病例产生的新病例低于1。用专业术语来说，就是需要将**再生数**——单个病例产生的新病例的平均数量——降至1以下。如果能做到这一点，那么这种疾病将从整体人群中消亡，即使有少数不幸的人仍会被感染。

再生数取决于疾病的生物学特性：它能以多快的速度产生15 新的感染性颗粒？这些颗粒在自然环境中的生存状况如何？再生数还取决于控制相遇筛选的宿主的生态和行为：群体密度有多大，宿主之间如何相互作用，以及它们相互作用的频率如何？最后，再生数还取决于疾病易感人群的比例，随着人们首先被感染，然后痊愈（通常来说，至少是暂时对该疾病免疫）或死亡，该比例在传染病流行的过程中会下降。为了忽略这最后一个复杂因素，流行病学家将重点放在**基本再生数**R_0上。R_0是指，在新发传染病疫情中，第一例感染病例所导致的病例数。R_0是衡量疾病生物学和群落结构的基本指标，它并不取决于流行病在人群中传播的程度。如果能关闭相容和相遇筛选，将基本再生数降低至小于1，那么不仅可以控制正在暴发的流行病，而且可以在第一时间防止疾病的发生。

罗纳德·罗斯最先意识到这种以平均水平为中心的群体层

面思维在疾病控制中的重要性，他建立了疟疾传播的数学模型，证明可以在不完全消灭蚊子的情况下，只将蚊子数量降低到一个临界值以下，即平均每个感染者传播不到一例新发传染病例，就可以根除疟疾。（正如第六章中所述，灭蚊和其他关闭相遇和相容筛选的方法，已经成功地在某些地区消灭了疟疾，但并不是在全世界范围内。）罗斯因阐明疟疾的生命周期在1902年获得了诺贝尔奖，但在诺贝尔基金会网站上，罗斯的传记写道："也许他最大的（贡献）是为（疟疾）流行病学研究建立了数学模型。"

罗斯创立的模型是最早的**仓室模型**之一，该模型根据疾病状态将人群分为不同类的仓室，并追踪患者从一种疾病状态转变为另一种疾病状态的变化率。最常见、最简单的仓室模型被称为**SIR模型**，它将人群分为**易感者**、**感染者**和**病愈者**。易感者是指可能被感染，但目前尚未被感染的人（即此类人群的相容筛选是打开的）；感染者是指患有疾病，并且可以传播疾病的人（即他们是**易传染的**，又是被感染的）；病愈者是感染过某类传染病，但暂时对该疾病有免疫力的人。

最初的仓室模型衍生出许多变种，例如，SIS模型代表淋病等疾病，一旦疾病治愈（比如服用抗生素后），由于没有有效的免疫力，患者就会直接回到易感区。很多书籍和数千篇科学论文都是关于仓室模型的。虽然仓室模型最初的版本非常简单，但后来研究者们又增加了各种复杂的内容，考虑了遗传、年龄和营养等因素对相容筛选的影响，并构建了各种社会和空间网络的模型来表现相遇筛选。仓室模型还建立了大型计算机模型的基本结构，可跟踪美国国民每个人的行为和感染状况，以了解流感疫情的空间传播。

虽然既定疾病的生物学事实的现实性和可信度很重要，但仓室模型仍然是流行病学建模的主要手段，因为即使形式简单，仓室模型也可以捕捉到疾病在人群中传播的大多数重要特征。特别是当我们对某一疾病的重要信息一无所知时——流行病学家对这种情况非常熟悉——只要我们谨慎地解释其结论，极度简化的模型可能比过于复杂的模型更有用。

仓室模型通常假设人群中每个人一开始对某种疾病的易17感性相同（在出生时，或者一旦性生活活跃，就会发生性传播疾病）。易感者以某种方式与感染者接触，从而被感染，例如，咳嗽、打喷嚏或交换体液。一般来说，感染率会随着感染者在人群中的比例增加而增加，但不同的模型之间的细节差异很大。疾病传播的**感染期**过后，感染者就会康复，进入病愈者仓室，获得对疾病的有效免疫力。正如我们所见，该模型可能有很多变数，包括按年龄、性别或地理位置对人群进行细分；允许人们在一段时间后从病愈者类回到易感者类；或者允许不同个体传播疾病的速度发生变化。

即使不涉及任何基础数学，SIR模型的结构（图1）也有助于对我们控制流行病的方法进行分类。最常见的控制策略是，通过免疫接种或**预防性**药物治疗（即仅预防而非治愈疾病的药物）关闭相容筛选，将个体直接从易感者仓室移至病愈者仓室中，而途中不经过感染者仓室。几乎所有其他流行病控制的措施都会以某种方式影响相遇筛选。对于野生动物或家畜和植物中的流行病，杀死易感或感染的个体（**扑杀**），可将这些个体完全从种群中移除，有望将R_0降至1以下。尽管争议不断，但扑杀是为数不多可控制牛口蹄疫病毒的有效策略之一。暴露后治疗提高了个体进入病愈者仓室的速度，重要的是缩短了感染期，减少了其可能感染的易感者数量。最后，隔离等控制传播的措施可以阻止感染，而无须在仓室间移动人员。 18

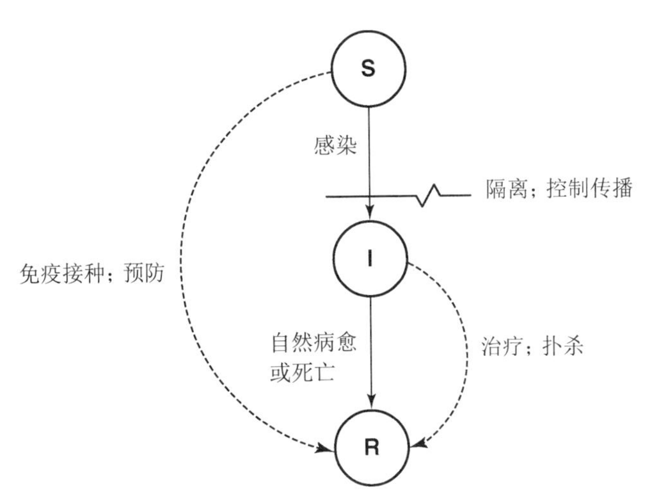

图1 SIR模型描述了人们从易感到感染再到病愈阶段的疾病发展过程。诸如扑杀、治疗或隔离等干预措施可以加速或防止仓室之间的转换。

除了考虑疾病控制措施的概念性框架外，SIR模型还提供了一个定量框架，可以准确地计算出根除一种疾病所需的控制量，或者给定的控制水平可以降低疾病水平的程度。假设我们可以通过关闭相容筛选（例如，接种疫苗）或相遇筛选（例如，提供安全套或干净的针头），通过**控制分数**（p）来消除部分有效接触。那么，R_0的值将减小$1-p$；如果R_0最初等于4，并且我们可以达到0.75或75%的控制分数，那么可将R_0减小为$(1-0.75)\times4=1$。

一些代数表明，为了将R_0降到1以下，我们需要将控制量增加到临界值$P_{crit}=1-1/R_0$以上（图2）。这说明了虽然天花和麻疹都有廉价且有效的疫苗，但为什么消灭天花（$R_0\approx6$，$P_{crit}\approx0.8$）

19 比消灭麻疹（$R_0 \approx 15$，$P_{crit} \approx 0.95$）容易得多，以及为什么即使有了有效的疫苗，消灭疟疾也极其困难：据估计，在某些地区，R_0大于100，因此临界控制分数将大于99%。实际上，在疟疾高发地区根除疟疾的唯一办法可能是将几种不同的策略（如疫苗和防蚊）结合起来，每种策略都可能（例如）达到90%的有效性，从而使综合效力能够达到需要的99%的水平。

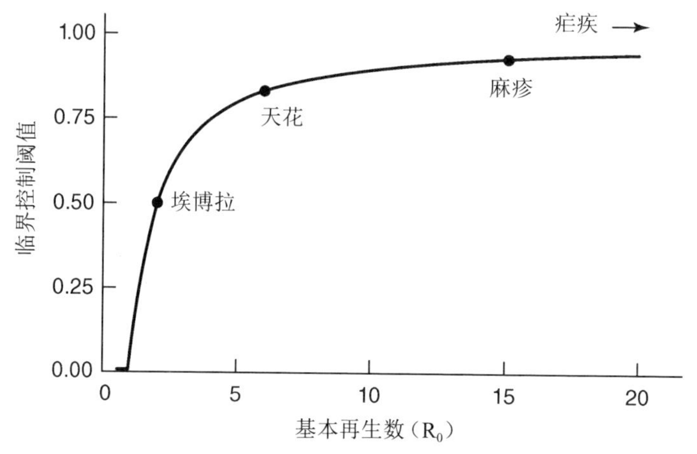

图2　根据传染病的R_0值，消灭传染病所需的临界控制水平（免疫接种或治疗以防止传播的比例）。

原则上，如果疾病控制措施能够将R_0降至1以下，不仅可以终止现有的任何流行病，而且只要维持控制措施，就可以防止疫情再次发生。在特定区域（如英国或欧洲），根除一种疾病，可以减轻当地传染病的负担，但并不能消除疾病控制的必要性，除非公共卫生当局能以某种方式百分之百地确定可以防止疾病从根除区域之外输入。只有当我们能够在全球范围内消灭一种疾

20 病时，才能安全地停止防控措施，但迄今为止就只对天花和牛瘟（一种与麻疹密切相关的致死性牛病）可以做到。这使得根除

而不仅仅是简单地控制一种疾病，成为一种有吸引力的政策选择——一旦疾病完全消失，用于防控它的任何资源都可以腾出来，分配给其他疾病的控制工作，或用于其他社会目标。

当然，了解R_0并不能告诉我们有关疾病防控的所有信息，例如流感（$R_0≈2—3$）和艾滋病（$R_0≈2—5$）等疾病要比R_0值相对较低的疾病更难以控制。有时无法治疗，或治疗费用过于昂贵。在其他情况下，治疗或控制措施仅部分有效。如果疫苗的有效率仅为50%，与目前正在测试的实验性疟疾疫苗相当，并且比现有效果最佳的HIV疫苗（≈30%有效率）更高，因此需要治疗的人数就是现在的两倍（如果$R_0>2$，这种疫苗就不可能根除该疾病）。另一个问题是，由于生物或文化原因，感染可能难以检测，因此无法控制疾病。从生物学角度来讲，某些人（携带者）被感染并传播疾病，却没有表现出任何症状；从文化上讲，许多疾病带有耻辱感，使人们隐瞒自己被感染的事实。在西非埃博拉疫情期间，实施严厉控制措施的主要问题之一是，这些措施可能只会鼓励有埃博拉接触史的人向政府隐瞒。

仓室模型远不止说明了局部地区或在全球范围内消灭疾病所必需的控制水平。模型还提供了一个简单的公式，计算在没有控制的情况下疾病暴发将影响的人数，或在人群中得到确认的疾病达到均衡时易感人群的规模。仓室模型也有助于流行病学家思考疾病的动态变化，即受感染人群随时间变化的方式。

例如，仓室模型的最早应用之一解释了，观测到的麻疹流行具有年周期性，并不一定意味着每隔几年就有一种新的基因型入侵；相反，疾病传播的速度快，会导致易感人群数量减少，需要数年时间才能达到引起另一次大规模暴发的程度。同样，数学家也指出，疫苗接种如果不能根除一种疾病，就会让人群中的易感者数量不断增加。即使疫苗接种覆盖率很高，这些增多的易感者可能会在接种的几年后导致大规模暴发。如果没有这种动态的洞察力，疫情很容易被解释为疫苗有效性或疾病传播性的突然变化，而不是亚临界控制水平的直接后果。

宿主传染病动力学

仓室模型在追求简单的过程中，忽略了许多生物学细节，其中之一就是缺乏对疾病在单个宿主体内传播方式的描述。在仓室模型中，宿主要么被感染，要么不被感染；我们既不跟踪人体内部的感染程度（例如，病毒感染的细胞数量或血液中病毒的密度），也不跟踪免疫系统对疾病的反应。

标准的仓室模型最适合于了解小型病原体（**微寄生虫**），如病毒、细菌和真菌；因为该类病原体往往在宿主体内能迅速积聚，并在大多数宿主中触发类似的免疫反应，所以将宿主描述为感染或未感染是一种合理的简化。在被**大寄生虫**，如绦虫或蜱虫等感染的人群中，每个宿主体内的寄生虫数量在个体之间有很大差异。

22

为了解释这种变化，数学家不得不设计更复杂的模型。然而，在过去十年左右的时间里，随着研究人员建立更精细的微寄生虫模型，跟踪感染颗粒或细胞数量的变化以及个体内免疫系统的激活水平，这些差异开始变得模糊。例如，HIV的传播大部分发生在感染后的第一个月内。如果想了解和预测HIV的流行，我们显然需要使用模型来区分新近感染者和非新近感染者；我们甚至可能想要追踪感染者血液和其他体液中病毒载量的精确水平。

嵌套模型既能追踪感染者数量的变化，又能追踪人体内被感染细胞数量的变化，但从数学角度而言非常复杂——可想而知，要追踪群体中每个人体内的所有病毒颗粒是多么困难！相对来说，宿主内模型更易于管理，该模型专注于疾病在人体内的发展，而忽略疾病在个体之间如何进行传播。流行病学模型可以描述疾病在人群中的发展，并深入了解疾病在群体层面的影响和控制，而宿主内模型则有助于了解疾病在个体中的作用方式。

然而，尽管范围有所不同，流行病学模型和宿主内模型有着惊人的相似性（图3）。仓室模型可以很容易地适应宿主内模型，特别是病毒等必须侵入宿主细胞才能进行繁殖的寄生虫。我们不再假设感染在单个宿主内迅速形成并且具有特异性，以便可以识别未感染或感染的宿主；而是假设感染程度（如病毒载量）在宿主细胞内迅速而特异性地加重。相遇筛选和相容筛选的概念 23

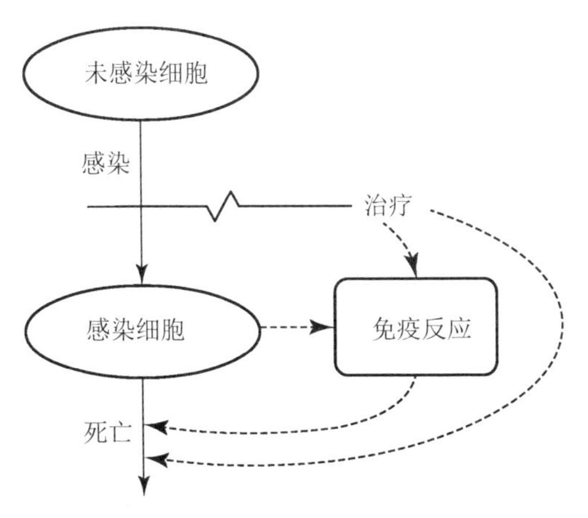

图3 宿主仓室模型表明：细胞的感染和感染细胞的死亡；感染细胞和治疗触发免疫反应；通过免疫反应和治疗杀死感染细胞；通过治疗阻断细胞间传播。

在宿主内和种群内层面同样有用，它们描述了感染是如何在细胞间传播，以及是什么阻止或允许疾病病原体感染细胞。

在宿主内模型中，通常会添加一个新的仓室来追踪细胞外自由浮动的感染性颗粒，并且有单独的术语来描述宿主内激活的免疫防御水平。在宿主内模型中，还通常假设免疫防御的强度随着受感染细胞数量的增加而增强。如果免疫反应足够迅速且足够强大，这些模型就能表明免疫系统是如何自然地战胜感染的，尽管不一定是在感染暂时扩散并感染另一个宿主之前。宿主内模型还可以阐明药物治疗如何能够充分减缓疾病在宿主体内的传播进程，使免疫反应足以消灭疾病。在攻击免疫细胞的病毒中，如HIV和人类T淋巴细胞病毒等，宿主内模型准确地显示了这些疾病如何颠覆正常的免疫策略；免疫系统通过激活更多的免疫细胞来对抗病毒感染，这反而为病毒的生长提供了更多的资源。这就像发现你正试图用汽油而不是水来灭火。

毒力、抵抗力和耐受性

仓室模型最常用于广泛传播的疾病，如麻疹、小儿麻痹症或天花，几乎所有人都对这些疾病易感。人类对感染的易感性确实存在差异：因为个体之间有不同的基因型（即全套遗传物质），或者营养状况有好有坏，或者压力的大小。疾病对每个人的传染性、患病后的严重程度以及致死性也各不相同。然而，对于流行病的防控规划而言，至少在疾病流行的初期，忽略这些细节差异是明智的。

但当我们考虑进化时，这种变化则不仅危险且不容忽视，而且对于我们提出的问题也至关重要。在过去的几十年里，流行病学建模专家已从试图了解疾病在几天到几年的时间范围内如何在人群中进行传播，转变为了解疾病在几年到数千年内如何演变的过程。特定宿主、特定寄生虫和特定环境的结合让寄生虫感染宿主的原因是什么？是什么决定了宿主被感染后是重症还是只有轻微的症状？

我们必须对寄生虫的特征做出几个重要的区分。首先是传染性（寄生虫感染宿主的难易程度）和毒力（寄生虫成功感染宿主后对其造成伤害的严重程度）之间的区别。我们通常将传染性和毒力视为寄生虫的固有特性。不管寄生虫或其感染宿主的基因如何构成，天花的症状远比麻疹可怕，致死性也更强。麻疹比天花的传染性更强，而天花比HIV或埃博拉病毒传染性更强。但原则上，我们可以想象到两种寄生虫菌株和两种宿主在作用上的“交叉”，其中一种寄生虫对第一宿主基因型的毒力高于第二宿主基因型，而另一种寄生虫则对第二宿主基因型的毒力更强。

25

宿主可以通过两种方式控制攻击它们的病原体的传染性和毒力。如果宿主能够部分或完全关闭相容筛选，则说明其可以抵抗寄生虫。因此，寄生虫可能根本无法感染宿主，或者其种群数量可能无法在宿主体内增加到非常高的水平，从而对宿主几乎不会造成不良影响。抑或宿主可能会被寄生虫感染（或者更确切地说，宿主可能不花费精力进行自身防御），但是它可以进化出一些机制，避免自身感染后受到严重损害：在这种情况下，我们称宿主对寄生虫耐受而不是抵抗。

在宿主个体层面上，耐受性和抵抗力有相似的结局（宿主不受寄生虫的伤害），但在群体层面上结局却迥然不同。如果某些人对传染病高度易感（既不抵抗也不耐受），那么具有抵抗力的人将有助于降低总体的感染机会，而耐受的人则会增加感染的机会。这也是流行病学家担心引入部分有效疫苗的原因之一。如果病原体进化成能更快地在宿主体内复制，以克服接种疫苗者的部分抵抗力，那么对于未接种疫苗的人，病原体的毒力可能会增加；如果接种疫苗使人们对疾病具有耐受性而不是抵抗力，那么病原体仍然可能感染未接种疫苗的人。

26

第三章

流 感

除非很幸运或很谨慎，每个人在一生中，都可能会感染流感。流感几乎尽人皆知，全球范围内每年都会出现。在历史的长河中，流感一直伴随着我们。虽然流感不像一些病毒性疾病如埃博拉那样可怕，但自14世纪黑死病（淋巴腺鼠疫）暴发以来，流感病毒造成的死亡人数超过了任何一次传染病暴发所导致的死亡病例数：1918年的西班牙流感造成全球2 000万到5 000万人死亡。

此外，虽然非流行病学家可能不认为这是一个大问题，但每年冬季在全球温带地区发生的流感疫情都会感染数百万人。尽管死于流感的仅为小部分体弱的老年人，但人们仍然认为，在美国，在流感流行的典型年份（不是大流行年份）会导致多达四万人死亡。由于流感会间接导致许多人死亡，例如引起继发感染，因此这些数字是在流感季节性大流行年份中，通过观察额外死亡人数而间接估算的。

流感在某些年份更为可怕，比如2009年，当时人们可能正处于一场致命性流感大流行的边缘，这场大流行可能导致数百万人而不是数万人死亡。流感大流行是在非常特殊的情况下27发生的，但最重要的两个因素是缺乏既有免疫力（相容筛选的漏洞）和毒力。如果病毒的外形发生了根本性的变化，则会有更多的人易受到感染，因为先前获得的免疫力无法抵御新毒株。这使得R_0（基本再生数，见第二章）的值高于病情严重的年份。如果病毒同时具有更强的毒性，重症患者比例会较往年更高，所以传染率增高是最可怕的。2009年政府部门担心上述情况有三个原因：（1）新毒株是H1N1型，与前一年的H3N2型不同，人们更易感并且R_0更高；（2）1918年的强毒性流感大流行是由H1N1毒株引起的；（3）由于墨西哥的报道有偏差，2009年流感病毒的毒性最初被高估了。

最后，虽然2009年的H1N1毒株对年轻人造成相对严重的影响，导致很多年轻患者死亡，但在整体上，其毒性与普通流感毒株相差无几。2009年的H1N1流感毒株引发了一场大流行，也就是说，一种此前未被观察到的病毒株在世界范围内导致了大量的感染病例，但可喜的是，它并没有像最初我们担忧的那样感染那么多人，也没有导致那么多人死亡。

为了防止大流行，我们必须控制疾病传播。传播可以通过减少接触（打喷嚏时用肘部而不是手掌遮挡口鼻）、减少相容性（接种疫苗，降低易感人群的数量）或最好是两者结合。在2009年的H1N1疫情中，相关部门采取了关闭墨西哥各地的学校，阻止大型公众集会，分发口罩和洗手液等措施，降低了接触率。研制疫苗能迅速关闭流感新毒株的相容筛选；H1N1疫苗于2009年10月上市，距H1N1毒株鉴定后仅六个月。上市初期，疫苗数

量有限，因此优先发放给最高危的目标人群，**以及**最有可能传播 28
H1N1的人群，包括学龄儿童。我们将在本章后文讨论为什么儿童是流感疫苗接种的重要目标人群。

在第一世界国家，注射流感疫苗（或者至少是疫苗的广泛宣传）和白昼缩短一样，预示着冬季的来临。与发达国家的公民在儿童时期接种过的麻疹或白喉疫苗不同，我们每年都需要注射新的流感疫苗，因为流感病毒进化很快；病毒外壳变化迅速，因此我们的免疫系统每年都需要找寻新的线索来识别病毒古老而熟悉的伪装。

理解流感的控制，有助于理解导致流感病毒独特的外形变化能力的进化过程。如第一章所述，宿主和寄生虫就像《爱丽丝漫游奇境》中的爱丽丝和红桃皇后：她们必须尽全力奔跑，才能保持在同一个地方。宿主和寄生虫处于一种竞争状态，宿主为了逃避寄生虫的入侵而不断进化，而寄生虫则为了跟上宿主的步伐而进行相应的进化。对于宿主来说，赢得比赛意味着关闭相容筛选，寄生虫就无法再利用它。对于寄生虫而言，获胜意味着保持相容筛选的开放状态，这样它就可以继续利用宿主。因此，“同一个地方”就意味着寄生虫仍然可以感染宿主；全力奔跑意味着宿主和寄生虫都在快速进化，宿主试图逃脱寄生虫的感染，而寄生虫则顽强地与宿主斗智斗勇。

重要的是要记住，进化并不总是通过自然选择，人们通常记住的是从学校课本上学到的“适者生存”范式。任何一个自然种群都包含许多不同基因型的生物体；种群中任一给定基因型所占的当前比例被称为**基因型频率**。对于进化生物学家来说，进化意味着随时间的推移基因型频率的**任何**改变。有关进化的

29 热点问题主要集中在自然选择的过程，基因型频率因适应度（即每个基因型的预期后代数量和存活概率）的不同而发生变化。但基因型频率也会因偶然事件而改变，这一过程被称为**基因漂变**。

为了进一步区分自然选择和基因漂变，我们可以假想一种传染病。假设宿主基因型发生随机突变，该突变对疾病具有完全抵抗力，并且没有副作用。如果这种疾病很常见，那么由于自然选择，人群中的这种突变频率应该会增加；携带突变基因的人在疾病发生的情况下会有更高的适应度，而在疾病不存在的情况下也会有同样的适应度。然而，在突变频率增加之前，有一个小概率事件，即发生基因突变的家庭成员很可能会一起出行，并在一次交通事故中全体丧生。这是基因漂变的一个例子：进化的发生是因为一个偶然事件，与传染病、宿主的适应度或突变本身无关。即使对于专业流行病学家来说，预测流感流行也极为困难，原因之一就是流感是通过基因漂变和自然选择而进化的；在温带流感季节之前发生的偶然事件，可能会让当年的流感疫情走上不同的、不可预测的轨道。

进化需要基因变异。基因变异的最终来源是突变，这是一种病毒擅长的过程。基因变异的另一个重要来源是重组，即基因以不同的方式组合现有的基因型。流感病毒就能利用突变和**基因重排**——重组的一种方式。如后文所述，宿主（即人类）通过突变进化的能力是有限的，但是我们能充分利用重组，将其作为免疫系统的重要特征。我们之所以能识别这么多寄生虫，并不是因为我们的基因编码了不同的蛋白质（**抗体**）来识别每一种
30 寄生虫，而是人类的基因组必须要比寄生虫庞大的基因组大

很多倍。相反，人类的基因能在不同的组合中重复使用相同的小片段基因来产生一系列抗体，不同的抗体可以识别很多不同寄生虫的特定部分，即抗原。

人类的基因组是由DNA组成的，DNA是由一种名为聚合酶的特殊蛋白质复制而来。DNA聚合酶不仅能复制DNA，还能校对产生的新链，并能纠正复制过程中许多不可避免的错误。流感病毒的基因组是用RNA而不是DNA编码的。RNA还编码自己的RNA聚合酶。然而，与人类用来复制DNA的聚合酶不同，流感病毒的RNA聚合酶不能校对以纠正复制错误。因此，流感病毒的复制最终会在新的基因组拷贝中出现越来越多的错误，即突变。由新的、突变的RNA基因组产生的病毒将会发生突变，其后代也会发生突变。其结果是，流感病毒基因组的突变率是人类基因组的十万倍。因为流感突变速度快，所以进化也很快。

流感病毒的突变会导致**抗原漂移**，这是流感病毒随时间的推移缓慢变化的过程。在抗原漂移的情况下，人体有时可以使用同一组抗体来识别已发生突变的流感毒株。打个比方，短袖衬衫的花色可能已经从条纹变成纯色再变成格子，但是不管花色怎么变，衬衫依旧还是衬衫。然后，由抗原漂移产生的新流感病毒会通过自然选择和基因漂变两种方式进化，因此这类流感病毒在逃避现有宿主抗体库的防御方面有更高的适应度。由于流感病毒不断进化，因此，无论是接种过流感疫苗还是有流感接触史但未接种流感疫苗的人，在几年后都会自然地失去免疫力。

流感病毒还有另一个进化的技巧，其基因组被分成八个不连续的片段，因此流感病毒可以将这些片段的不同变体重新组

31 合，产生新型病毒。当流感病毒的两种不同变体恰好侵入宿主内的同一细胞时，它们可以重新排列，彼此交换基因组片段，产生**抗原转移**。这种重组导致病毒外壳发生快速且戏剧性的变化，有效地将“短袖衬衫”换成了“夹克”。人体的免疫系统难以识别这些变化，所以流感病毒打开了相容筛选。因此，重组病毒的子代具有进化优势，并且如果它们更易感染宿主，克服相遇筛选，则会在种群中传播。

抗原漂移通常不足以引起大流行。但大流行流感的标志是抗原转移，尤其是在多个宿主中发现重组流感毒株。例如，2009年的H1N1流感是起源于猪，这些病毒的不同基因片段能整合至鸟类、人类和猪的基因组。

流感病毒不断变化的外壳由来自两个独立基因的蛋白质组成，即血凝素（HA）和神经氨酸酶（NA）。流感毒株是根据每个基因的变异命名的：H1N1结合了HA变体#1和NA变体#1。当一种特定的流感毒株将其HA和NA基因换成另一种类型时，我们的免疫系统就不能，有时甚至完全不能识别流感病毒。HA和NA是抗原，是人体的免疫系统识别寄生虫的部分。这些抗原暴露在病毒颗粒的表面，当它们漂浮在血液中时，我们的免疫系统可以检测到它们。当病毒感染细胞时，它们会把细胞变成生产更多病毒的工厂；当出现流感时，新病毒是通过“出芽”的方式从细胞中冒出来的，而不是完全使细胞分裂。作为出芽过程的一部分，被感染的细胞在其表面显露HA和NA，从而触发免疫系统识别和破坏所选择的细胞。32

流感疫苗主要有两大类。标准三价流感疫苗（TIV）是一种肌肉注射的灭活或“被杀死的”病毒。另一种是新型、应用较少的疫苗，市面上名为FluMist或FluEnz，是一种减毒（弱化）但“活的”病毒（LAIV）的鼻腔喷雾剂。（这里的“被杀死的”和“活的”加了引号，因为生物学家的共识是病毒不是活的生物体，但“活的”和“被杀死的”这两个词仍然被普遍使用。）这两种疫苗都含有三种不同的毒株，这些毒株预计在即将到来的流感季节会很常见。有时，如果相同的毒株仍然很常见，则连续几年流感的发生都可能与其有关，但疫苗研发人员通常也会研究至少一种新型毒株来预测抗原漂移或转移。

TIV和LAIV均可触发人体最常见的抗体——免疫球蛋白G（IgG）的反应。IgG对漂移可能引起的相对细微的变化很敏感。换句话说，如果注射液仅包含带有“条纹”的病毒，并且发生了突变，让其外壳变成“纯色”，则免疫系统将无法检测到已变化的病毒——更不用说病毒由于抗原转移而产生的更复杂变化，例如将“T恤”换成“休闲夹克”。正是由于IgG对于HA和NA差异的处理能力相对有限，再加上抗原漂移的持续过程，我们每年都需要重新注射新研发的疫苗。

LAIV还会触发人体免疫系统的其他部分，如免疫球蛋白A（IgA）和细胞介导免疫（CMI）。IgA是另一种存在于血液和黏液中的抗体。CMI是一种独特的免疫类型，这种免疫类型不涉及抗体，而只负责杀死人体内被病毒利用并转变成病毒工厂的细胞。通过破坏病毒产生的途径，而不仅仅是清除血液中的病毒颗粒（见图3），CMI可能比抗体介导免疫更有效。

如果LAIV这么有效，为什么没有得到更广泛的应用呢？主要有两个原因。首先，最重要的一点，TIV在成人体内产生的免疫反应更有效——较强的IgG反应要优于较弱或缺失的IgA/

CMI反应。其次，注射LAIV的人可以在疫苗接种后的短时间内释放病毒（即将病毒释放到可以感染他人的自然环境中）。免疫力较弱的人，与刚接种疫苗的人密切接触，是有感染风险的。不建议免疫力低下人群接种LAIV，包括孕妇、两岁以下或四十九岁以上者，以及患有艾滋病等慢性感染疾病者。

现代疫苗接种计划不仅旨在保护个体，而且还为了保护群体。疫苗可以通过多种方式减缓每年流感流行的严重程度。首先，疫苗可以完全预防接种者受到感染。这能显著降低感染率——不仅能保护疫苗接种者，而且保护了可能被病毒感染的每个人。然而，即使疫苗不能完全阻断感染，但也可以减少后续的传播。接种过TIV的成年人，即使不幸感染了流感，通常也会比没有接种疫苗的人恢复得更快。患者能从中获益（症状持续的时间更短，有助于更早返回工作岗位）；疫苗也降低了总体感染率，因为接种者在其缩短的感染期内传播给他人的机会更小。病毒在体内存活期间，接种疫苗的人也可能排出更少量的病毒，因此传染性也较小。最后，疫苗接种者通过群体免疫帮助控制疫情（见第二章）：（从病原体的角度来看）感染者与疫苗接种者的潜在传染性接触是无效的，这会导致R_0下降。如果有足够多的人（超过$1-1/R_0$的比例）能进行免疫接种，那么感染者每人所造成的新感染病例将少于一例，病毒将趋于灭绝。

重要的是确定优先接种对象，特别是在疫苗供应有限的情况下，如2009年H1N1暴发初期的情况。即使有足够的疫苗，公共卫生机构也必须明确目标人群，进行针对性的疫苗接种宣传和推广。重点为最有可能罹患严重疾病或死亡者进行接种。然而，在这类群体中，很多人正是因为免疫系统功能低下而发生不良事件，这意味着即使能够说服他们接种疫苗，也可能无法保护他们。另一种补充办法是着重为最有可能传播病毒的人接种疫苗。

流行病学家使用接触网络来识别人群中传播率高的个体。接触网络关注的是传播的“相遇”阶段——如果未感染者没有接触感染者，传播就不会发生。图4显示了美国一个由父母、两个孩子和一个祖父组成的中产阶级家庭。一位家长在外和其他三位同事做小生意，另一位家长在网上做生意，并和生意伙伴在当地的咖啡店工作很长时间。这两个五岁和七岁的孩子在当地的小学上学。每个孩子都有十个同学加一个老师。祖父独立生活，但住在家附近，每周都会来家里吃几次饭。

35

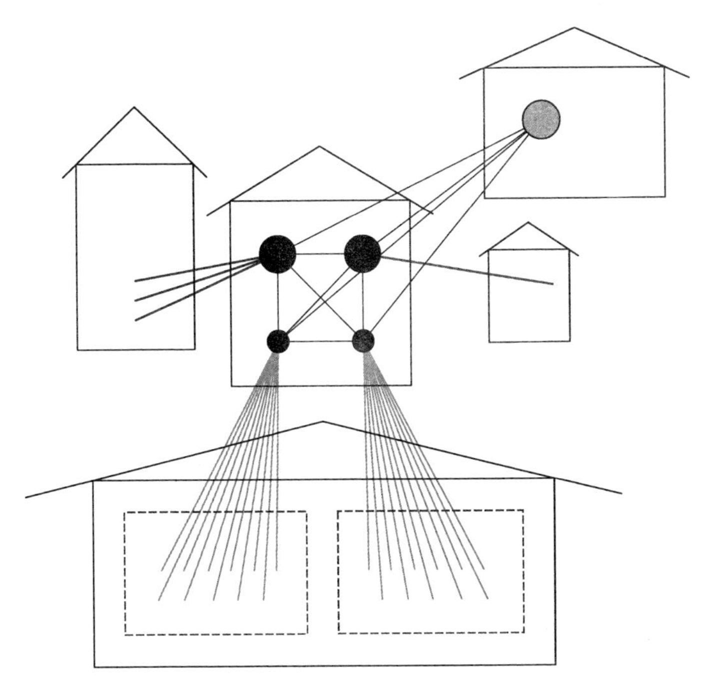

图4 西方中产阶级家庭的联系网络，由父母、两位学龄儿童和独立生活的祖父组成。

与人打招呼等不经意的交往，偶尔才会导致流感的传播。流感最重要的传播途径是经常性的身体接触，或是打喷嚏和沾染上别人打喷嚏时产生的飞沫。每一次这样的接触，对于核心家族中的每一个成员，都会在图中用一条线表示。这个简化（但并非不切实际）的例子表明，儿童在流行病学上有意义的接触次数最多。可想而知，孩子是最有可能将疾病传染给家庭成员的人，尤其是传染给祖父，他最容易出现流感并发症。因此，为儿童接种疫苗是当务之急，这不仅是为了保护他们，也是为了保护老年人。显然，地区之间的接触网络以及地区之内的社会经济地位差异很大，因此需要进行认真的比较工作，以确定全球疫苗接种的优先事项。

流感也是一个有意思的案例研究，它阐述了一个古老的争论：某些研究是否因太过危险而不允许开展？如果的确要继续进行这项研究，那么研究结果是否仅提供给有限的、经过严格筛选的研究人员和政策制定者，还是应该对所有人开放？

科学研究由政府组织、非政府组织和产业界资助。产业研究通常是归个人所有，是私有的，这样公司就可以获得投资回报。但政府和非政府组织资助的研究是为人民服务的科学。这类工作的成果应所有人可见，特别是当研究最终由税收和慈善捐款资助，并直接与人类健康相关时。

不幸的是，一些有助于预测流行病的研究也可能被生物恐怖分子不法利用。此类“双重用途”的研究受国际条约和出口限制的约束。即使没有故意滥用，如果实验室研制的超级病毒株意外流出研究实验室，也可能发生可怕的事情。

流感大流行的最关键指标是传播途径——这决定了禽类、

36

猪或人类的HA和NA类型的新组合会否在人群中广泛传播。只有在人与人之间进行有效传播，特别是通过空气传播，流感才会构成大流行。因此，一个重要的公共卫生优先事项是了解人与人之间的空气传播是如何进行的，以及我们应该寻找哪些可识别的标志来提前检测新出现的大流行病毒株，以防止它们广泛传播。

21世纪的前二十年，拥护知识民主化者与担心知识滥用者因有关流感的研究产生了对峙。隐藏在这项有争议研究背后的主要动机很简单：如果我们能够理解是什么样的基因变异使大流行流感不同于常规的季节流感，就有可能预见导致大流行病毒株的产生，并采取适当的预防措施，特别是哪些变异导致通过空气传播。由于资源有限，而且我们重视个人自由及公共健康，因此无法对每种流感做出最大反应。因此，只有在风险很高的情况下才应采取特殊的防控措施，但是我们怎么知道何时超过该阈值呢？

37

流感研究从2011年开始备受关注，不是因为在了解流感流行方面取得了突破，而是因为两篇关于空气传播的高调论文的发表引发了争议。科学家们正在研究一种毒性极强的禽流感毒株H5N1，如何在雪貂之间通过空气传播。雪貂是研究流感病毒在人类中传播的重要动物模型系统，部分原因是雪貂和人类一样，在感染流感时会打喷嚏。

这项研究的发表之路漫长而坎坷。论文最初是在2011年8月提交的。四个月后，美国国家生物安全顾问委员会最初建议在这两篇论文中省略实验的关键细节，以解决安全问题。2012年5月，在文章接受两个月后，第一篇论文终于在网上发表。第二篇论文于同年6月下旬发表，并被流行播客《本周病毒播客》讽刺地称为“第二只雪貂的启示”。一旦国际专家们认定，发表论文的潜在公共卫生利益，包括所有细节，都超过了潜在的危害，论文才可以未经审核地顺利发表。

这场争论有一个特别有意思的地方，2012年冬天，科学家们自己同意暂停对H5N1病毒的**功能获得性**研究——制造出高危流感病毒——直到可以讨论有关问题和采取适当的保障措施。2012年的禁令最初被提议持续六十天，但最终持续了将近一年。这种自我强加的限制很少见，但对维护公众对科学的信心至关重要。然而，2014年10月，美国政府发布了一项新的暂停令，禁止资助关于功能获得性的新研究，这不是因为担心生物恐怖主义，而是因为美国政府的关键研究中心错误地处理了其他病原体的潜在危险样本。

38

“两篇著名但近乎未发表的论文”发现，HA是与流感病毒外壳进化相关的最重要的两种物质之一，它决定了特定流感毒株的传播能力和毒性。例如，某些形式的HA，如存在于H1N1病毒中，就可以通过我们鼻部和咽喉部细胞表面的蛋白质感染人体细胞。这类病毒具有很强的传播性，不需要深入人体体内，就可以轻易地感染新宿主。但H1N1病毒的毒性并不高，因为病毒通常不能发现适宜的细胞而感染肺部深处，因此很少导致肺炎等相关疾病。但其他形式的HA，如H5N1，则只入侵肺部深处合适的细胞。因此，这类病毒会损害肺部，导致肺炎，因此毒性更强。然而，这种危险病毒株的传播率很低，因为H5N1病毒颗粒除非能够深入人体肺部，否则无法造成感染。

多亏了已发表的关于雪貂的研究，我们知道只需要少量的突变，H5N1就可以进化出在人群中进行空气传播的能力，至少研究人员所研究的H5N1病毒的特定毒株具备这样的能力。此外，H5N1毒株哪些基因发生了突变已经很明确。我们已经确定了这种特殊病毒株在大流行前病毒外壳可能会发生的变化，因此在流感大暴发前就能识别它。如果在所有能进行空气传播的39病毒株中都发现了这些特征性突变，就可以通过追踪家禽和人类流感病例样本的基因序列，来检测流感何时会变成空气传播（因此可能会大流行）。

为什么要对“这种特殊的病毒株”提出警告？因为流感病毒的进化，就像其他病毒进化一样，取决于从哪种病毒株开始。虽然我们知道，研究人员研究的H5N1特定毒株可能引发流感大流行，但我们不知道是否可以将这些想法应用于H5N1的其他病毒株，更不用说像目前在亚洲流行的H7N9这类不同的毒株了。

不管一个人对“两篇著名但近乎未发表的论文”的智慧或实用性有何看法，它们都开启了未来双重用途研究的先河。科学家在决定是否发表这项研究时所展示出的克制表明，科研界以及世界各国领导人可能最终采纳了预防性原则（在任何负面结果发生之前进行审查，而不是在事实发生之后进行审查）。这也表明，科学家们意识到，广泛的利益相关者积极参与研究，对于维持公众对科学的信任至关重要。40

第四章

HIV

我们的第二个传染病案例研究是HIV，一种可能为大多数读者所熟悉的病毒。HIV是一种人类免疫缺陷病毒，会导致获得性免疫缺陷综合征，即艾滋病。感染了HIV后，感染者可能会携带病毒长期生存而不会出现任何症状，但是仍然能够传播HIV。在初次感染一段时间后（通常是几年），感染者体内的病毒数量开始迅速增加，最终导致免疫系统崩溃。于是，HIV阳性者就很容易受到由能诱发肺炎的**卡氏肺孢菌**或**白色念珠菌**等病原体所造成的机会性感染（见第二章）；免疫系统功能正常的人通常不会感染这两种病原体。艾滋病患者也更易罹患某些类型的癌症，如卡波西氏肉瘤。未经治疗的HIV感染通常在五到十年内致命。死亡的直接原因通常是机会性感染，而不是HIV本身。

HIV是一种与流感截然不同的病毒；它在个体之间有着不同的传播方式，也有着不同的进化潜能。HIV往往在人与人之间最亲密的时刻通过体液交换而发生传播。许多人认为HIV主要是一种性传播疾病，因为精液和阴道分泌物携带的病毒均足[41]以引起感染。然而，人体血液也携带HIV，这意味着，当接触到感染者的血液时，任何人都可能被感染。医务人员不慎被针扎伤，静脉吸毒者共用针头。输血者，特别是血友病患者和其他需要频繁输血的患者，往往在HIV流行的早期就受到感染（现在大多数血液供应品都进行了严格的HIV和许多其他血液病原体的筛查）。由于母乳也会携带病毒，所以感染HIV的母亲可在哺乳期将病毒传染给婴儿。

了解传播途径是保护人群和个体的关键，人们可以因此相应地改变自己的行为（安全性行为，针对静脉吸毒者的针头更换方案，针对卫生工作者的眼部保护和针头扎伤治疗方案等）。如后文所述，确定最常见的传播途径，也有助于合理使用有限的HIV治疗资源。但是，在我们了解治疗方法之前，需要更多地了解HIV。

HIV带来的最大挑战之一是其有强大的进化能力。人们认为，HIV有一层隐形的斗篷，而不是像流感一样披上了一系列款式相似的外衣。在最初几十年里，有关HIV的研究举步维艰，因为HIV有一种让人匪夷所思的能力，能逃避人体免疫系统的监视，治疗效果也所见甚微。我们无法研发出HIV疫苗，因为该病毒的进化速度太快了——比流感更快，而流感病毒外壳通过数年的进化已经发生了翻天覆地的变化！这种进化的能力也意味着HIV在全球范围内发生了惊人的变异。因此，在研制疫苗时，我们要追踪的不仅仅是一个动态靶点，而是很多靶点。我们担心永远无法研发出一种具有持久疗效的药物，因为HIV似乎不费吹灰之力就能让药物失去作用。那么，要想研究HIV，就必须[42]

明确这种致命消失行为的作用机制。

HIV的隐匿性部分源于一种“阴险”的逃逸策略：它隐藏在人类自己的基因组中。HIV是一种逆转录病毒，这意味着其自身有一个RNA基因组，它首先可以通过一种复杂的病毒蛋白——**逆转录酶**——被复制进DNA中。由此产生的双链DNA可以通过另一种病毒蛋白——**整合酶**——整合到人类基因组中。事实上，HIV成为人类身体里的一部分，这也是它难以治愈的原因之一。

然而，HIV只能侵入特定类型的细胞，这是第二章中所述的相容筛选的一个例子。细胞必须有表面蛋白（受体）来与HIV包膜外的一个特殊的“旋钮”gp120（糖蛋白，一种分子量为120的糖类蛋白质）相结合，HIV才能进入细胞。因此，阻断gp120相容筛选可能会有效抵抗HIV。值得注意的是，在人类基因组中可能存在一种突变，能实现上述功能。HIV实际上需要结合两种受体才能进入细胞：gp120的主要受体（被称为CD4）和辅助受体（被称为CCR5）。具有CCR5-Δ32突变的人群缺少gp120的共同受体，因此对HIV的感染具有抵抗力。然而，要想完全避免HIV感染，必须有这种突变的两个拷贝，每个DNA链上都有一个。但具有CCR5-Δ32（杂合子）单拷贝的人仍可被感染并出现症状，尽管与完全没有拷贝的人相比，他们对HIV有更强的抵抗力。

人体只有三种细胞有合适的受体与gp120结合，这三种细胞都是我们免疫系统的一部分。正是因为HIV的靶细胞是免疫细胞，所以感染HIV后会导致免疫缺陷。病毒隐匿在这些免疫细胞中，直到它被激活。一旦被激活，病毒就开始复制，最终导

致免疫细胞死亡，并削弱人体对抗其他感染的能力。 43

如第三章中有关流感的描述，突变是随机发生的，与病毒是否发生有利进化无关。因此，病毒的突变率对于了解突变发生的难易程度（以及发生的频率）至关重要。凭直觉来说，我们可以预期HIV的突变率要比流感病毒高得多，因为它进化很快。HIV的突变率确实比流感病毒高出十倍以上。

有趣的是，对HIV突变率的估算在很大程度上取决于具体情况，例如，人体中和试管中的病毒，突变率大有不同。

HIV的复制需要两种不同的酶。一种是病毒自身的逆转录酶，如前文所述，它将病毒RNA转化为DNA。而已经整合到人类基因组的病毒DNA会通过第二种酶，即人体自身的RNA聚合酶进行复制。于是，这些新的RNA基因组被重新包装成病毒颗粒，从细胞中释放出来感染另一个细胞。大多数HIV的突变来自病毒的逆转录。HIV逆转录酶比被流感病毒所用的酶更易出错，因此HIV的突变率高于流感病毒。

突变并不是HIV变异的唯一来源。与流感不同的是，流感病毒的基因组是分段的，因此来自多个病毒的不同基因片段可以结合在一起，而HIV则是将其单基因组的片段与其他HIV病毒的基因组片段进行交换，这一过程被称为重组。然而，HIV的重组与人、果蝇或豌豆等生物体的基因重组有着本质上的区别。当RNA中的信息被复制进DNA中时，基因就在逆转录中发生了重组。病毒的逆转录酶有时会从一种模板（被复制的病毒基因组）转换到另一种模板（如此往复），这一过程被称为模板转换。为了理解模板转换，可以想象你在描绘纸上描摹两条平行 44 线，但一次只允许描摹一条直线。从左端开始，向右移动。可以想象，描摹纸随机上下移动，交替描画顶部的线和底部的线，但始终从左向右绘制。最后，绘制成了一条直线，但它包含了两条直线各部分的拷贝。同样，重组的HIV基因组包含单个基因组的所有部分，但由两个不同的拷贝重组而成。

突变和重组让HIV不断地进化，甚至逃脱了人们的监视。如前文所述，由于疫苗依赖于免疫学上对病原体靶点的免疫“照相记忆”，因此，如前所述，研发HIV疫苗非常困难。但是，HIV的隐匿性可能是其使药物无用的惊人能力当中最臭名昭著的，因其能在宿主体内快速进化出抗药性。

前文已探讨了人类的突变基因CCR5-Δ32，该突变通过阻断相容筛选而对HIV产生抵抗力。事实证明，在HIV流行之前，这种突变就已经在人群中存在了。虽然发现HIV感染人类只有一个世纪左右的时间，但在人类遗骸的DNA中已经发现了CCR5-Δ32突变。因此，我们有直接证据表明，CCR5-Δ32突变已经存在了近三千年。由于HIV的出现较CCR5-Δ32突变早得多，并且后者在某些群体中普遍存在，因此研究人员推测，CCR5-Δ32突变出现的频率较高，是因为该突变可以避免人类感染一些古老的传染病，如鼠疫或天花。然而，对CCR5-Δ32基因及其邻近DNA的仔细分析表明，如今这种高频率的突变很可能是一次令人欣喜的意外——这是基因漂变而非自然选择的结果。其他不太为人所熟知的对HIV具有抵抗力的基因似乎也比HIV更早出现。45

与人类基因组中的抗药性突变不同，虽然抗药性病毒株有时会在人与人之间传播，但HIV的抗药性往往是由于人体内新的病毒突变引起的。尽管面临着这些挑战，但在20世纪90年代中期，一种**高效抗逆转录病毒疗法**（HAART）问世了，这种方法可以非常有效地对抗HIV。高效抗逆转录病毒疗法联合了三种药物，能抑制HIV的增殖。一般说来，这些药物以两种不同的方式直接阻断HIV逆转录。一类药物的作用是通过诱导逆转录酶，结合化学物质，阻止RNA基因组的延伸。这些化学物质类似于逆转录的构建模块，但功能不同。一旦这些化学物质之一被整合，逆转录酶就不能继续合成基因组。这类药物被称为**核苷逆转录酶抑制剂**；高效抗逆转录病毒疗法中通常使用两种不同的核苷逆转录酶抑制剂。另一类药物直接与逆转录酶结合，使其无法发挥作用。这些药物被称为**非核苷类逆转录酶抑制剂**；通常在高效抗逆转录病毒疗法中只使用一种非核苷类逆转录酶抑制剂，来补充核苷逆转录酶抑制剂。

HIV产生对非核苷类逆转录酶抑制剂（例如）抗药性突变的可能性微乎其微。然而，如果有机会发生，即使对于个体来说不大可能发生的事件，也可能变得常见。单个HIV在人体内的存活时间并不长：血液中的HIV病毒在人体内的存活时间约为六个小时。因为病毒的总数大概是恒定的，这就意味着人体内的病毒每天大约会更替四次。此外，每一个感染了HIV的人，体内都有成千上万个病毒。因此，病毒每隔几天就会产生数亿次的复制周期，因而也就有了突变的机会。我们可以用彩票来比喻：如果你买了数亿张彩票，最终大概率会中大奖。换言之，由于感染者体内有大量的病毒，并且病毒进化速度很快，所以即使小概率产生的突变，最终也会发生。

46

高效抗逆转录病毒疗法的效果为何显著，需要记住两点：第一，突变是随机发生的；第二，独立事件同时发生的基本概率法则。要想抵抗高效抗逆转录病毒疗法，HIV需要有三个独立的突变基因，三种药物都需要相对应的突变。因为突变是独立的，在同一个人身上发生的机会是每种突变独立发生的概率的乘积。也就是说，如果每个事件的概率为0.5，那么两个此类事件的概率为0.5×0.5，三个事件发生的概率为0.5×0.5×0.5。现在想象一下，每一个个体突变的概率都远小于0.5。我们面对的不是“极不可能”，而是“极不可能的三次方”，因此，如果可以的话，即使有数千万种病毒和数亿个复制周期，抗药性的出现也需要很长时间。

抗逆转录病毒疗法曾经只是完全型艾滋病患者的治疗方案，部分原因是抗药性问题和资源有限。然而，2013年，世界卫生组织宣布了一种振奋人心的新型治疗模式：“治疗即预防”。根据这一战略，受感染但一般情况良好的患者也将接受治疗，从而减少病毒传播。与未接受治疗的人相比，接受药物治疗的患者，体液中循环的病毒更少，因此传播病毒的可能性更小。就个人而言，接受治疗者将在更长的时间内保持更健康、更快乐和生产力。有些人甚至可能永远不会出现症状。

然而，高效抗逆转录病毒疗法只是一种治疗手段，而不能达到治愈。患者需要每天服药，否则病毒载量又会增加，因为如前所述，病毒的拷贝隐匿在人体的细胞内，不受药物的干扰。事实上，中断治疗会很快导致病毒数量反弹到治疗前的水平。为了完全治愈HIV感染，我们必须杀死体内所有的细胞，因为这些细胞的基因组已在不知不觉中成了HIV的避风港。由于含有病毒整合拷贝的三种类型的细胞都是从骨髓中衍生出来的，实际上，临床医生已经在尝试有策略地破坏及替换骨髓，就像针对如白

47

血病这类癌症所做的一样。

首先，化疗是用来清除所有可能感染HIV的细胞，即使有些细胞可能没有被感染。但是，这也就破坏了组成免疫系统关键部分的细胞，如果没有这些免疫细胞，我们将无法长期生存。因此，下一步就是将未感染者的骨髓移植到患者体内，从而产生新的、未受感染的免疫细胞。同时，为了防止新产生的免疫细胞受到感染，在整个化疗和移植过程中，都采用了积极的抗病毒疗法来杀死当时在血液中循环的病毒。

一位名叫蒂莫西·雷·布朗的艾滋病患者，在接受治疗四年多后，仍无法检测出病毒。然而，另外两名患者中，治疗后的一年内HIV就达到了可检测水平。患者之间的情况并不完全相同：布朗接受了一名捐赠者的移植，这名捐赠者携带两个CCR5-Δ32的拷贝，这种突变可以通过阻断gp120相容筛选而产生抗HIV的能力。其他患者接受的移植，只有一个拷贝。他们的新骨髓对HIV感染只有部分抵抗力。

遗憾的是，由于捐赠者和受捐者之间的骨髓很难匹配，因此，要找到一个骨髓匹配的捐赠者，并且有两个CCR5-Δ32拷贝的可能性很小。仅仅因为这个原因，骨髓移植不可能作为一种艾滋病的普遍治疗方法。此外，移植手术需要长期住院进行治疗，因此数百万HIV感染者中的大部分人都不适合此种治疗方法。然而，蒂莫西·雷·布朗被治愈的意义是巨大的，他被成功医治无疑将激发出可以更广泛使用的治疗方法。例如，该疗法突显了CCR5-Δ32突变的重要性，它有可能推动以基因突变为基础的新疗法。 48

在HIV研究和一般传染病研究中，一个迫在眉睫的问题是

“为什么是现在”？HIV是从哪里来的，它是如何迅速对人类健康和经济稳定构成全球性威胁的？如果我们能解答这些问题，可能就能更好地预防其他新发传染病或减缓发病情况。

研究人员用两种主要工具来解释HIV的出现：接触网络（在第三章中讨论过）和系统进化树。系统进化树是进化生物学的基本工具之一，它是一种按相似性对生物进行分组的方式，而这种方式又可以通过相关性进行分组（如果深入研究）。图5展示了HIV和流感的系统进化树。如今，大多数的系统进化学都是利用基因信息构建的。两种生物的共同祖先越近，它们的关系就越密切，基因组也就越相似。我们使用系统进化树来显示

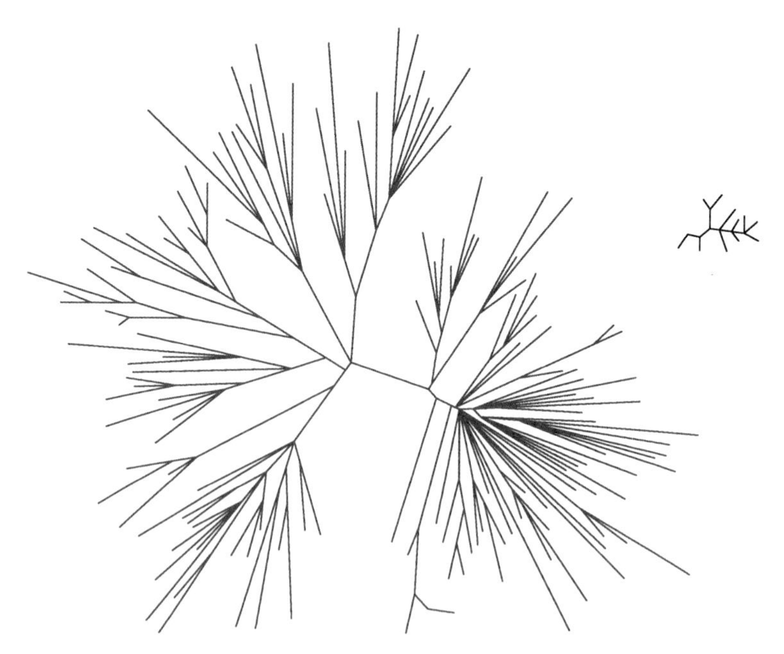

图5 HIV（左图，较大）的特点是在任何特定时间内都有广泛的基因变异，病毒株会长期存在。流感病毒（右图，较小）的特点是在任何特定时间内变化不大，而且随着时间的推移，病毒株之间会发生替代，而不是共存。

49

亲缘关系，将在系统进化上关系更密切的基因组放在一起，而将关系较远的基因组放在较远的地方。我们建立系统进化树的能力再次依赖于基因组突变的随机性（和相对恒定的速率）：基因组相似性是以两个生物之间不同的突变数量来评估的。但是，我们用系统进化树可以做的不仅仅是了解亲缘关系。我们建立系统进化树，是因为通过分析系统进化树的形状，可以了解在什么时间跨度上发生了什么样的进化过程。

如果突变在密切相关的物种中以相似的速度发生——几乎总是如此——那么我们可以简单地通过计算突变的数量来估计时间。如果两个病毒相差七个突变，比起两个变异类型相同的病毒（例如，具有二十个突变），它们的亲缘关系更密切，而且拥有共同的祖先。在系统进化树上，分支的长度与突变数量成正比，因此与时间成正比。

然而，系统进化树中除了树枝的长度，还含有很多有用的信息：树的形状也可以告诉我们很多关于病毒进化的信息。将流感树与HIV树进行比较，可以让我们立刻有一个直观的认识。流感树的树上有几根靠近树干的短枝。这种形状表明大部分流感病毒在人群的存活时间并不长，至少出现频率不高。随着流感的暴发，新的突变病毒迅速占领种群，取代旧的毒株。HIV树则要复杂得多。因为有很多长长的树枝，所以很难确定核心树干。与流感病毒不同的是，HIV的新突变体往往会与旧的病毒株长期共存，同时进化，但又是独立发展的。

最合理的推测是，最初感染HIV的患者，可能是因为食用了已经被HIV感染的黑猩猩。但是，为什么**现在**HIV会构成大流行呢？ HIV的原始病毒SIV已经存在了数千年，因此人们很可

50

能与它接触了很长时间。当代的病毒和小心储存在医院冷藏室的旧的血液样本的系统进化树表明，最广泛流行的HIV-1的M型病毒起源于1910年至1930年间，虽然最初的人畜共患病（病毒起源于黑猩猩）可能更早出现。其他不太常见的HIV-1的型式是独立起源的，在某些情况下，可能比M型的起源更早，但这样也在同一时间增加了流行率。是不是当时发生了什么事情导致了现在的大流行？

要解答这个问题，我们首先要理解病原体从非人类宿主传播给人类的过程（人畜共患病，见第一章）。人畜共患病有两种典型的传播方式：一种是人畜共患病在人群中的R_0小于1，即每位感染者引发的新发感染例数不足一例，这被称为溢出事件。个别感染者可能罹患重病或死亡，但由于疾病在人与人之间的传播率非常低，以至不会真正发生物种间的跳跃转移或宿主转移。另一方面，如果R_0略大于1，即持久性的最小值，那么病原体就可以成功地转移宿主。一旦病原体开始在人与人之间传播，就可能发生突变，以适应新的宿主。换句话说，这些突变会把相容筛选越开越远。

51

如前文所述，突变是随机的，突变的概率也是随机的。突变的概率与可突变的基因组数量成正比。因此，在人畜共患病流行初期快速采取应对措施，通过降低人类感染病例数来限制总的突变率至关重要。例如，2003年，美国暴发了西半球首次猴痘疫情，原因是宿主通过非洲冈比亚袋鼠将猴痘病毒传播给圈养草原狗，而草原狗又在宠物交易中将病毒传播给了人类。在非洲，猴痘病毒在人与人之间的传播中至少已经进化了一次（也有可能是多次）。但是，由于感染者很快得到了医治，加上医疗机构卫生状况良好，美国猴痘病毒在人群中的传播没有发生变异，疫情期间仅出现了71例病例，无死亡病例。

目前，解释当前HIV大流行最简单的观点是，病毒不会进化，只是我们运气不好。根据这一观点，SIV感染人类（经相遇筛选）并发生传播（打开相容筛选）的概率，不会随时间而发生改变；20世纪初暴发的疫情是病毒进化最成功的一次。无论何时，宿主转移成功的概率很低，但SIV与灵长类宿主及人类已经长期共存，所以HIV在黑猩猩与人类之间的传播以前不可能没发生过。

关于HIV的起源，目前的主流观点是，灵长类动物的确多次把HIV传播给人类，但因为HIV从未超出最初的感染范围传播，所以没有引起世界其他国家的注意。（埃博拉病毒也发生了类似的传播过程：小规模疫情可能在部分人群中持续了几个世纪或几千年，并在过去四十年里有所记录。2014年，随着它在西非城市中的出现，西方国家才开始密切关注。）然而，最近一次HIV转移到人类时，恰逢人类的人口学和社会学发生变化，从而促进了传播。这种特殊的宿主转移恰好与非洲的城市化进程相吻合，而城市化建设已经持续了一段时间，而修路又将许多与世隔绝的地区连接起来。此外，政治动荡、性革命和全球流动性的增加也与宿主转移相吻合。

52

其他研究人员则认为，像受感染黑猩猩的血液通过伤口进入人体这类简单的生物学事件，尚不足以触发一次人畜共患病的转移，而在进化为适应人类的HIV的道路上，SIV在无意中得到了人类的帮助。重复使用未经消毒的注射器，医疗操作也可能与病毒在人体中持续存在有关，直到人与人之间传播的病毒发生突变。两种假设——城市化和使用未经消毒的注射器——并不矛盾，而且还很可能协同作用于病毒的传播。我们永远无法确定，但通过追问HIV的来源，我们吸取了重要的经验教训，53 这些经验教训已经被用于遏制其他病原体传播的防控中。

第五章

霍　乱

在任何关于传染病的讨论中，霍乱都具有一种基础性的作用。霍乱引发了流行病学的支柱之一——科赫假设。该假设指出，要确定某一特定的病原体是某一疾病的致病因素，需要满足以下条件：（1）患者体内有该病原体，而健康者无。（2）可从患者体内分离出病原体并进行培养。（3）实验室培养的病原体感染新宿主后会致病。（4）病原体可以从新感染的宿主体内重新分离出来。霍乱也使人们认识到，预防措施应以供应清洁水源为重点，这一举措，能关闭其他大量水媒病原体的相遇筛选。

霍乱弧菌是引起一种名为霍乱的腹泻疾病的病原体，它是一个庞大且类型多样的菌种。根据一个特定样本能否与哺乳动物感染已知类型时所产生的抗体发生反应，新的样本被分为不同类型。这种抗体具有很强的特异性，只与能在哺乳动物体内产生抗体的霍乱弧菌发生反应。故这些抗体可以被用来鉴别不同的霍乱弧菌菌株。因此，如果新型菌株与注射了O1型菌株的动物所产生的抗体发生反应，则该菌株也是O1型。这些抗体被

54 称为**血清型**，意思是“基于血清的类型”，因为抗体是从血液（或血清中）分离出来的。两种血清型，即O1型和O139型，是导致大多数霍乱的罪魁祸首。即使是这两种血清型的霍乱弧菌，也只有在携带至少两种特殊基因的情况下才能引起流行病：一种是克服相容筛选，另一种是打开相遇筛选。

当摄入大约一百万个霍乱弧菌时，人才会感染霍乱弧菌。胃酸除了有消化食物的功能外，还能杀死我们不慎摄入的各种微生物，包括霍乱弧菌，以保护人体健康。食物有中和胃酸的作用，在完全空腹的情况下，需要一百万亿个霍乱弧菌才能被感染，比摄入食物时致病所需的细菌多十万倍。细菌数量庞大，有些细菌可以在胃酸的考验中存活下来，并顺利通过小肠。

胃酸中的细菌也必须能够感染小肠细胞才能致病。至少，霍乱弧菌必须有参与产生毒素共同调控菌毛或TCP的相关基因。TCP是相容因子的重要组成部分，没有它，就不会致病。许多其他基因都能增强定殖能力，但TCP是唯一必不可少的基因。值得注意的是，甚至在定殖后，除非霍乱肠毒素（CT）的基因被表达，否则霍乱弧菌通常也不致病；也就是说，霍乱弧菌具有传染性，但没有毒性。霍乱的毒力与传播力密切相关，CT对霍乱在宿主间的传播（其退出策略）至关重要。CT破坏了肠道的水分调节，引发宿主的严重腹泻，甚至导致脱水和死亡，但在腹泻后，霍乱弧菌能重新回到自然环境中，感染新宿主。

虽然霍乱的临床症状让人不寒而栗，但它的优势是治疗方55 法非常简单。服用含糖和盐的口服补液剂，就可以大大降低霍乱患者的死亡率，甚至完全避免死亡。虽然抗生素有效，但仅作为一种辅助防御手段（第二道防线）。抗生素最重要的优点就是缩短了传染期，从而降低了传播的风险。

霍乱在流行病学史上扮演了重要角色。斯诺发现了霍乱是由一种传染性病原体传播的疾病，并在19世纪中叶伦敦霍乱暴发期间，将病原体的栖身之地定位在一种特定的水泵上，这可以说是流行病学作为系统性侦测工作的第一个案例。

斯诺的观点在今天仍然有用：通过净水和建立水处理厂来关闭相遇筛选，是预防霍乱流行的绝佳策略。然而，靠煮沸来净化水（一种低技术含量的解决方案，可以在偏远地区或欠发达地区实施，能有效防止霍乱流行）需要大量的木柴，在政治不稳定的地区获取木柴可能很危险，并可能导致乱砍滥伐。采用高科技净水技术，价格昂贵，如处理厂或通过化学试剂净化水，而且在后勤方面可能略有困难。近年来，有一种操作简便、效果良好的净水新技术，是利用四种厚度的纱丽布过滤水，该技术可将感染率降低50%。

然而，即使建立了污水处理系统，感染者也会在自己家庭内部传播霍乱。霍乱的社会网络分析结果表明，感染在家庭内部的传播速度要比家庭之间的传播速度快得多，这很可能是由于家长手上携带的霍乱病原体污染了水或食物。因此，公共卫生机构推广了带有窄口和水龙头的储水容器（不是传统的开放式水桶），细菌携带者就不能把手或衣服浸入水中而污染家庭用水。这些干预措施使霍乱传播率降低了近40%。

霍乱弧菌是如何进化的？在与宿主的竞赛中，细菌的外观发生完全进化的频率低于病毒。由于细菌的生化机制与人类的大相径庭，故我们可以通过利用其他有抗菌效应物质的生物，如真菌等来抵御细菌（第一章）。但这种方法对于抗病毒来说基

56

本上是无效的，因为病毒利用人体内多种生化途径进行繁殖，在消灭病毒的同时，也会损害我们自身的健康。造成这种差异的另一个原因是，细菌的变异速度比病毒慢很多，单个细菌产生的突变不能快速累积，因而无法逃避人体免疫系统的监视。所以，细菌的进化主要依赖于抵抗宿主的抗菌策略。

霍乱弧菌的进化方式并不是更换整个“衣柜”，而是根据特定时间内的自然选择来获得（和丢失）“配饰”（对策），从而“装扮”自己。如果自然选择需要一条羽毛围巾，并且在服装包装盒（即当地环境）里正好有一条，那细菌只要选择它，就能繁殖。也就是说，带有羽毛围巾的细菌将比没有的细菌繁殖更多的后代，这就是通常意义上的自然选择。但是，对于细菌来说，甚至连羽毛围巾也很沉重，所以，如果不是明确的生存所需，放弃它对细菌的繁殖来说是最有利的。

细菌不戴围巾，但它们会获得或者丢失基因。新基因有两种来源途径：首先，可以从其他细菌中获取可移动的基因元件；其次，可来源于感染细菌的病毒。由于涉及不同代次而非亲代之间（纵向）的基因移动（横向），这两种机制都被称为横向基因转移。与哺乳动物的繁殖方式不同，细菌通过分裂进行繁殖，但横向基因转移并不需要产生新细菌或病毒，只需接触已有病原体即可。

57

我们最喜欢的实时进化的例子之一是细菌的抗生素抗药性，这通常是通过质粒上携带的基因（从染色体上分离出来的小环状DNA片段）由横向基因转移而来的。霍乱也不例外。虽然治疗霍乱不需要抗生素，但抗生素确实可以缩短传染期，缓解症状。大量使用抗生素会产生选择性抗药的情况。

与病毒不同的是，细菌的抗药性一般不会因为新的突变而产生，原因有以下几点。首先，如前所述，细菌的突变率通常比病毒的突变率低——这降低了细菌进化出新的抗药机制的能力。其次，与病毒相比，细菌更有可能在同代之间进行基因交换，即参与由横向基因转移。细菌中最臭名昭著的两个抗药案例是抗甲氧西林金黄色葡萄球菌（MRSA）和一种新型危害——抗碳青霉烯肠杆菌（CRE），是由于对不同种类抗生素抗药的基因引起的。

霍乱主要是通过获得一种叫作SXT的DNA片段而产生抗药性，这种DNA类似于质粒，但呈线性而不是圆形。一旦产生了抗药性，只要使用抗生素，细菌就比未产生抗药性的细菌更不易被杀灭。然而，当抗生素停止使用时，抗药性就会丧失。基因组大的细菌比基因组小的细菌需要更长的复制时间，因此，在没有抗生素的情况下，含有大量整合抗生素抗药基因的细菌，比没有这些基因的细菌复制时间更长。在快速增长的人口中，这可能是一个重要的障碍，被称为**抗药性的成本**。

就像DNA可以整合到基因组中一样，抗药基因也可以再次脱离基因组。如果出现这种情况，基因组较小的细菌可能会有优势。或者，如果抗生素抗药性基因在质粒上，而未在染色体上，如果质粒本身没有赋予细菌任何优势，那么它们可能会通过基因漂变而随机丢失。在其他细菌系统中，抗药性的成本可能是由抗药性基因的代谢成本所产生，这可能会使机体消耗大量的能量而将毒素泵出细胞，或者因为机体切换到对抗生素免疫但新陈代谢作用效率较低的生化途径。

霍乱弧菌在人体内寄生，病毒同时也能寄生于霍乱弧菌内。

58

值得注意的是，如前所述，细菌可以从病毒性寄生虫体内获取有用的基因，但发生概率较低。自然选择会奖励机会性生物体，因此在某些情况下，给宿主提供有用信息的病毒比不提供的病毒生存期更长。要清楚在什么样的情况下，霍乱弧菌会从病毒中获取新基因，我们必须进一步了解感染细菌的病毒：**噬菌体**。

常见的噬菌体是温和噬菌体，其有两种侵袭细菌的策略。第一种是溶原策略，即噬菌体一旦进入细胞，其DNA就被整合到细菌的基因组中。噬菌体的DNA被称为**前噬菌体**。前噬菌体与细菌自身的DNA共同复制，传播给初始受感染机体的所有子代。这是一个和平的王国，除非噬菌体得到生化信号，表明它已受到威胁。在这种情况下，噬菌体可以非破坏性地退出，或者它可以采用裂解策略。

在裂解策略中，噬菌体将细菌宿主转变为病毒工厂，子代繁殖到一定数量，就可通过裂解细胞来杀死细菌。新噬菌体又可以根据环境条件追求溶原或裂解策略继续感染其他细菌。

59

如前所述，只有少数霍乱弧菌菌株携带毒素基因CT。CT是温和噬菌体CTXφ送给宿主的礼物。一旦霍乱基因组中发现了CTXφ，毒素就能被表达并增加霍乱弧菌的传染性（从而增加R_0）。但是噬菌体，即使是温和噬菌体，也不是无私的。CT可以提高细菌的适应度，但同时也可以提高（现在）原噬菌体的适应度，并与患者肠道内的细菌共同繁殖。

导致霍乱大流行的另一个重要基因是TCP，如前所述，TCP能使霍乱弧菌在小肠定殖。TCP还有另一个功能，即它是噬菌体CTXφ的受体。受体是病毒宿主相容筛选的一部分。如果病毒和受体之间没有正确匹配，就不会发生感染。霍乱通过表达

TCP，引起CTXφ的感染，从而收到CT的礼物。这是一个既美丽又险恶的共同进化的例子：霍乱广泛传播所必需的两个组成部分（即原噬菌体的组成部分），是一个相互依存的系统的一部分，确保双方的健康。

但这种邀请和礼物的漂亮场景，是对更应被准确地看成一场持续恩怨的深刻误读。不管有没有礼物，细菌都不希望噬菌体来参加聚会，即使噬菌体退出也会给细菌施加一种成本，不管成本有多小。相反，噬菌体是一个聚会的破坏者。它把TCP作为受体，因为TCP是细菌自身需要的东西。而且CT也不是礼物。噬菌体携带它，只是因为它能增加噬菌体的适应度。如果噬菌体的适应度能随细菌的增加而增加，那很好，但之所以能这样工作，是因为噬菌体被整合到了细菌的基因组中，所以它们的适应度是密不可分的。但是，如果出现突变或新的DNA片段，就会以牺牲细菌为代价，进一步提高病毒的适应度，或者允许细菌在保持CT的同时摆脱其他破坏聚会的原噬菌体，自然选择会优化这种变化，所有礼貌社会（上流社会）的幻想都将会破灭。 60

事实上，有证据证明这个故事有更黑暗的版本。深入研究后，研究人员已经了解到，编码CT的基因很可能是噬菌体近期获得的。有许多相关的噬菌体没有携带CT，但仍然使用TCP作为它们的受体。此外，CT基因的组成表明，CT基因比基因组的其他部分要更新。不仅仅是细菌，寄生在细菌上的病毒也可以为了自己的利益而入侵。

为什么TCP没有进化，导致CTX噬菌体无法利用它，特别是因为许多这些噬菌体甚至都没有携带CT？ 噬菌体感染可能不会对霍乱细菌造成太大伤害，即使受到威胁，这种噬菌体也会不杀死细胞就离开它。因此，细菌通过改变TCP来抵抗感染的选择压力很小，特别是考虑到它们需要TCP到肠道定殖。

其他感染霍乱的噬菌体的行为更像是传统的掠食者，总是杀死猎物。这些噬菌体必须是裂解噬菌体；它们只能通过溶原或裂解它们的宿主来生存。换句话说，如果它们感染细菌，那注定会失败。这些裂解噬菌体中最著名的就是JSF噬菌体群。它们使用与CTXφ不同的受体进入霍乱细菌。

在霍乱肆虐的地区，霍乱的流行是有季节性的。科学家们最近注意到，恒河三角洲地区的霍乱疫情，往往是在水中的裂解噬菌体数量较少时开始，而在裂解噬菌体繁殖增多时结束。此外，霍乱患者体内噬菌体的相对丰度，也反映了其在水生环境中的相对丰度：在霍乱流行初期，患者体内的裂解噬菌体较少，而在流行后期则较多。上述结果表明，裂解噬菌体可能会在霍乱流行的基础上继续流行，甚至可能有助于控制霍乱的流行。

61

噬菌体可以在个体和群体层面控制霍乱。噬菌体疗法早在20世纪20年代就已经出现，该疗法最初用于治疗痢疾，痢疾是一种与霍乱类似的腹泻性疾病，但是由不同的细菌引起的。噬菌体疗法的最大优势在于，许多噬菌体对细菌具有特异性：没有副作用。常规抗生素不仅会攻击有害细菌，还会攻击人体内的必要细菌；很多女性都有遭受酵母菌感染的痛苦经历，因为抗生素杀死了她们生殖道内的常居菌群。设计良好的噬菌体疗法可以成功杀死有害细菌，而不会影响有益细菌。

噬菌体疗法的缺点是，噬菌体会试图利用有进化能力的生命系统。噬菌体一旦进入患者体内，它们就可以在自然选择的作用下，通过任何方式进化，包括可能致病的方式，例如CT。限制治疗性噬菌体与宿主细菌的基因整合能力，能在一定程度上降低这种治疗风险。在过去的六十年里，尽管很少有报道涉及噬菌体疗法的不良事件，但噬菌体的可进化性可能是噬菌体疗法在除俄罗斯和格鲁吉亚以外国家和地区没有被接受的原因之一。噬菌体疗法在世界范围内重新引发人们的兴趣，一部分是由于抗生素抗药性的增强，但也有部分原因是裂解噬菌体对在群体层面控制霍乱的流行成效显著。

霍乱流行的季节性值得深入研究。在孟加拉国，寄生在霍乱弧菌上的噬菌体也出现季节性波动。这些波动追踪霍乱密度的轨迹，似乎是以生态学家所熟知的常规（动物—动物或动物—植物）捕食者—猎物系统的模式：猎物（霍乱弧菌）首先增加，62 然后捕食者（噬菌体）增加，导致猎物再次减少。一旦猎物减少，捕食者缺乏食物，当然也会减少，这使猎物再次增加，形成多物种间的循环。因此，与其说是噬菌体控制了猎物，即霍乱弧菌的丰度，不如说是猎物促进了捕食者的丰度。对这一观点的支持来自这样的观察结果：海地的霍乱疫情也表现出季节性，但自然环境中几乎没有噬菌体。因此，季节性可能是由两地不同的发病机制引起的，或者噬菌体季节性是细菌季节性的结果而不是原因。

与人们对霍乱弧菌是通过饮用水传播的预期相反，霍乱弧菌是在盐水中生长的。如果水温适宜，并且营养物质含量丰富，霍乱弧菌也可以在淡水中存在。孟加拉国霍乱的流行与表层海水温度密切相关，原因有二。首先，海水表层温度的升高与强暴风雨有关，而暴风雨又会引发洪水。洪水能使已有的卫生问题恶化，将饮用水和污水混合，并加快了霍乱的传播。

其次，温暖的海面（特别是富含营养物质的海面）是一种名为浮游植物的微小植物大量繁殖的温床。浮游植物是浮游动物（微小的漂浮海洋动物）的食物。霍乱弧菌会黏附在虾类浮游动物的外骨骼上，这些浮游动物被称为桡足动物，它们的身体是由一种叫作甲壳素的物质组成的。人摄入大量的霍乱弧菌后，仅少数能在胃酸中存活。一只桡足动物体内约有一万个霍乱弧菌：食用桡足类就像吞下一颗霍乱炸弹。如果一只携带霍乱弧菌的桡足动物进入充满食物的胃，就可以轻易地传播足量的霍乱弧菌而致病，而饮用只含少量游离菌的水，则不会引发霍乱的传播。桡足动物身体上黏附了大量霍乱弧菌，这一点能解释霍乱的暴发起源于环境，而不是由感染者引起的。

63

与大多数重要的科学领域一样，关于霍乱的记录只有部分被科学界广泛接受。例如，霍乱弧菌依赖其生长环境的不同而表现出不同的感染情况，一直令科学家感到困惑。实验室中培养的霍乱弧菌是估算感染剂量（引发霍乱所需细菌的数量）的标准，然而，当志愿者摄入实验室培养的霍乱弧菌感染了肠道后，随腹泻排出的细菌会转变成**高传染性**。高传染性细菌致病所需的感染剂量更低。如果不援引这种高传染性状态，很难解释霍乱为什么能如此不可思议地迅速在人群中传播。例如，在1991年秘鲁霍乱流行的第一周就导致了三万例感染病例。

高传染性霍乱弧菌进入另一个宿主的肠道后，它仍旧处于高传染状态（只要它不被裂解噬菌体杀死，或不被抗生素击中）。另一方面，如果霍乱弧菌离开感染者的肠道并进入水中，但在五到二十四小时内未传染给他人，它就会发生另一种根本性的生理变化，变成一种截然不同的状态：“能活的但不可培养的”或“活跃的但不可培养的”。争议已显而易见：尽管人们已经认识这种现象三十多年，但我们甚至无法就如何称呼它达成一致！不可培养的霍乱弧菌作为新霍乱暴发的潜在环境宿主而备受关注。但这个过程是否可逆，特别是细菌进入不可培养状态后，是否能恢复它们在人类体内定殖的能力，目前尚无结论。 64

霍乱的另一个环境贮藏库，可能来自细胞进入水中后呈现的持留表型。当霍乱弧菌缺乏营养时，如离开人体肠道进入水源时，部分细胞可能会进入这种持留状态。与不可培养状态一样，持留状态似乎涉及休眠，并涉及基因表达和形态的变化。然而，持留菌是可以培养的，并且已经被实验证明，当资源足够时，特别是甲壳素，持留菌可以重新苏醒。

海地的霍乱疫情表明，了解霍乱暴发的源头和基因本身的毒性至关重要。2010年海地地震的悲剧因霍乱的暴发而加剧，在霍乱肆虐的第一年就报告超过47万例感染病例，其中6 631人死亡。海地至少有一百年未出现过霍乱确诊病例，这就直接提出了霍乱是如何传播的问题。从血清分型，到简单的比较特定基因的存在和缺失，再到复杂的系统发育分析，各种分析结果都表明，这些菌株并非来源于墨西哥湾等当地环境。

相反，从海地霍乱患者体内分离出的菌株与造成东南亚地区霍乱的菌株最为相似，这表明霍乱菌株可能是与来自东南亚地区的人或最近访问过该地区的人一起抵达的——在本次疫情中，霍乱菌株是来自尼泊尔的联合国维和人员。此外，维和人员的营地位于阿蒂博尼特河的一条支流上，虽然霍乱迅速蔓延到全国各地，但该河被确定为海地疫情的源头。 65

第六章

疟　疾

疟疾可能是世界范围内最重要的传染病。与前几章讨论的传染病相比，疟疾对温带发达国家的人来说不那么可怕——不是因为它的传染性或毒性较低，而是因为目前其传播受到蚊媒生态环境的限制，疟疾很少传播到热带地区以外。与霍乱不同的是，疟疾通常是地方性疾病——发病率在人群中长期保持在相对稳定的水平，而不像其他流行病一样突然暴发。作为典型的地方性疾病，传播最广泛的疟原虫通常会引起慢性感染且毒性较弱，并不会造成急性感染和死亡。但恶性疟疾是一个例外，这种类型的疟疾最常发生于热带的撒哈拉以南非洲地区。慢性疟疾导致的营养不良和贫血与儿童教育成效低下有关，而急性疟疾可导致慢性神经系统问题。从所有疟疾类型共有的对人类的非致命性影响与恶性疟疾的致命性影响结合来看，疟疾对人类的累积影响是巨大的。

公共卫生官员会利用**伤残调整寿命年**（DALYs）来衡量慢性病对人类的影响，它既考虑了疾病造成的生命损失，也衡量了

生产力和幸福感的损失。适当的权重显然会带来道德挑战。患 66
有慢性致残性疾病的患者生活一年是否相当于健康生活的六个月？三个月？一个月？应该如何比较死亡或残疾对婴儿、中年人或老年人的影响？然而，DALY的计算说明了一个事实，即疾病对患者的慢性影响可能与疾病导致的死亡同样重要，甚至更重要。2010年，疟疾造成的DALY损失比其他传染病都要严重，仅次于HIV/艾滋病。虽然很难得到确凿的证据——贫穷的国家往往是疟疾肆虐，而富裕的国家则鲜见疟疾病例，但研究人员表示，消除疟疾可使经济增长率提高几个百分点，这是挣扎中的经济和健康的经济之间的区别。

虽然每一种传染病都有其独特和神秘的地方，但疟疾比我们目前所讨论的传染病更加复杂。疟疾是由原生动物引起的，原生动物是一种单细胞生物，其遗传物质（与细菌不同）是在细胞核内。它的基因组由含大约2 300万个碱基对的DNA组成，比HIV和流感病毒基因组大数千倍，比霍乱弧菌的基因组大五倍左右。

疟疾的复杂性还源于其**病媒传播**的性质；疟疾通过不同种类的**按蚊**在人与人之间传播。霍乱可以调整其生化特性，交替作为海洋中的自由生物和人类肠道中的病原体进行传播。而疟疾则面临一个更具有挑战性的问题；它会根据两种不同的生物环境（人类宿主和蚊媒），以及每种宿主体内的多个器官（人类的血液和肝脏；蚊子的肠道和唾液腺）调整其生化特性。与物理环境相比，生物环境对寄生生物来说是更大的挑战。干燥和紫外线对寄生虫在宿主体外的物理环境进行传播是严重威胁， 67
但它们是被动的。相对来说，宿主机体会采取主动措施，通过免疫防御系统攻击寄生虫，从而消灭寄生“搭车者”。

感染人体的疟原虫常见的有四种类型。按所致疾病的严重程度由重到轻的顺序依次为**恶性疟原虫**、**间日疟原虫**、**卵形疟原虫**和**三日疟原虫**。（疟疾种类被称为**疟原虫属**，简称疟原虫及其种名。）第五种是**诺氏疟原虫**，其所引起的疾病在最初被认为是一种猕猴疾病，在东南亚正逐渐发展为人类的疾病，但迄今为止，只观察到猴对人（通过蚊子）的传播，而未发现存在人与人之间的传播。

所有疟原虫的生命周期基本相同。疟原虫首先在蚊子宿主的肠道中进行有性繁殖（雌、雄**配子体**的融合，相当于卵子和精子的融合），之后在下一个生命阶段（**子孢子**）游走到蚊子的唾液腺，并在蚊子叮咬人体时，将疟原虫注射进入宿主体内，以获得蛋白质来喂养它的卵子。（只有成熟的雌性蚊子才会叮咬人类，这对疟疾控制具有重要意义。）注射的子孢子侵入人类的肝脏，并进行简单的分裂繁殖，再迁移至血液，并随着种群的增长继续繁殖，感染和破坏红细胞。最终，疟原虫在血液中发育成雌、雄配子体，等待另一只雌蚊子的到来并吸取它们。

疟疾能通过破坏红细胞而引发贫血。然而，当疟原虫（最常见的是**恶性疟原虫**）进入大脑，导致脑型疟疾时，就会出现最严重的症状。在脑型疟疾中，寄生虫阻断血流并引发炎症，未经治疗的患者最终可能死亡，即使是治疗后康复的患者，也常常造成脑损伤。疟疾最明显的症状是发热，虽然发热本身似乎对人体的危害不大。随着新一波寄生虫从肝脏进入血液，发热会以特定频率反复出现：在历史上，疟原虫株就是根据每隔一天（**间日疟原虫**和**卵形疟原虫**）或每隔三天（**三日疟原虫**和**恶性疟原虫**）

复发来分类的。在许多疟疾流行地区，因为检测费用昂贵且需要专业知识，因发热和头痛来医院就诊的患者会自动接受疟疾治疗。

疟疾不能直接在人群中进行传播，这让疟疾的防控有了更多的可能性。如第二章所述，疾病模型的创始人之一罗纳德·罗斯发现了有关疟疾的两个重要事实。首先，他发现蚊子可以传播疟疾，这首次使通过灭蚊或防止蚊子叮咬（关闭相遇筛选）预防疟疾成为可能。其次，他的模型表明，公共卫生机构不需要彻底灭蚊来根除疟疾——只需要减少蚊子叮咬的次数，让平均每个疟疾感染者都不被蚊子叮咬，从而不引发新的感染病例。相遇筛选不需要完全关闭——只需适当关紧，以致只有几只蚊子能够潜入即可。

如果不能通过杀死、阻止或驱赶处于任一生命阶段的蚊子来关闭相遇筛选，则可以尝试关闭相容筛选。在史前时期，人类进化出许多关闭相容筛选的遗传机制，不过通常是要付出代价的。甚至在人类尚未清楚疟疾的病因之前，我们就已经研发出了药物来阻断相容筛选，即通过在人体内，以对人类的毒性比对疟疾的毒性小一些的方式对抗疟疾。例如，从19世纪初开始，由于在汤力水中发现奎宁的抗疟作用，金汤力就成为热带地区英国殖民者最喜欢的饮料。近年来，研发人员着力于研制疟疾疫苗，以期增加人类的自然免疫力，尽管到目前为止尚未完全成功。接下来，我们将讨论这三种相容阻遏策略。

生物学家从四千年前的埃及木乃伊中提取了古老的DNA，但疟疾在此之前就已经存在。早在一亿年前，人们就在藏身于琥珀中的蠓（咬人的苍蝇）的内脏中发现了疟疾的近亲，这些蠓

69

很可能会叮咬冷血爬行动物。然而，这种化石极为罕见，为了解决一亿年前到三千年前的差距，我们必须求助于疟疾及其宿主的基因组。

疟原虫属于一个庞大而复杂的家族——顶复门原虫，它经常在宿主之间跳跃。虽然蜥蜴、鸟类和哺乳动物体内的疟疾寄生虫都被称为疟原虫，但它们很可能是两个独立的科（一个感染蜥蜴和鸟类，一个感染哺乳动物），并且与其他寄生虫的关系比彼此更密切；大约在一千三百万年前，哺乳动物的疟疾就从顶复门原虫家族的其他物种中分离出来。感染人类的疟原虫是混合群体；它们与非人类宿主的各种疟原虫的关系都比彼此更密切，这些疟原虫大约在二百万到七百万年前分离出来。

究竟是哪个非人类宿主，在何时开始传播人类疟疾，是一个迅速发展且有争议的话题。恶性疟原虫是造成人类疟疾最危险的一种疟原虫，其基因组的分析表明，在大约一万年前，随着农业的发展和人口密度的增加，恶性疟原虫的数量显著增加。恶性疟原虫的来源仍是一个更棘手的问题。尽管它与引发黑猩猩疟疾的疟原虫关系紧密，旧版教科书中指出，恶性疟原虫是由黑猩猩传播给人类的，但最近的两项研究提出了新颖而矛盾的说法。第一项研究在圈养倭黑猩猩（黑猩猩和人类的近亲）的血液样本中发现了关系更密切的疟原虫；第二项研究在野生大猩猩的粪便中发现了与恶性疟原虫关系更密切的虫株。但这些结果仍然存在争议。大猩猩研究的作者指出，在野生黑猩猩和倭黑猩猩中，与恶性疟原虫相关的感染很少见，因此倭黑猩猩感染最有可能来自人类。不管探究恶性疟原虫真正起源的结论如何，结果都表明，我们对疟疾、疟疾宿主及其病媒的复杂生态系统所知甚少。

人类基因组进一步地揭示了人类与疟疾相互作用的历史。人体并不是疟原虫的温床；我们的免疫系统不断进化出新策略来对抗疟原虫的破坏性影响。人类有多种遗传性抗疟疾策略，其效力和副作用的严重程度各不相同。其中最典型的是镰状细胞。生物学教科书中描述了镰状细胞通过杂合子优势来抗疟疾的例子：携带一个镰状细胞等位基因和一个正常血红蛋白等位基因的人对恶性疟疾有部分耐受性，但携带两个等位基因的人则会罹患严重的镰状细胞贫血。

地中海贫血是另一种与镰状细胞贫血类似但由基因突变引发的疾病，在地中海地区相对较常见。该突变通过修改红细胞来减轻疟疾的严重程度，但会导致贫血。葡萄糖-6-磷酸脱氢酶（G6PD）缺乏症在地中海地区发病率也很高，该病可预防恶性疟和间日疟。G6PD也可导致贫血，但仅在特殊情况下，例如食用蚕豆或服用常见的抗疟药，比如氯喹或伯氨喹。达菲阴性，即缺乏“达菲抗原”，这是一种帮助间日疟原虫和诺氏疟原虫靶向进入红细胞的蛋白质，虽然能预防疟疾，但有很多并发症。

71

遗传分析可以预估突变发生的时间长短。我们熟知的人类O型血似乎能预防疟疾，但O型血很古老，它已经存在了数百万年，比疟疾出现的时间还要长，因此其早期进化可能是抵御另一种目前未知的血液病原体，但不是预防疟疾。达菲血型抗原阴性的部分变体大约有三万年的历史。G6PD缺乏症在五千至一万年前就已存在，这加强了恶性疟原虫基因组的证据，即随着农业的发展，恶性疟疾给人类带来的风险激增。相比之下，一些镰状细胞变异体进化时间很短，只有几百年或几千年的历史，这提醒我们，人类和疟疾基因组在不断（共同）进化。

由于这些基因保护机制同时会引发严重的并发症，自然选择只在疟疾流行风险高于产生副作用风险的地区增加其频率。在其他地区，自然选择会降低其频率。由于疟疾传播范围广，而且会产生致命的影响，自然选择可能是过去几千年来塑造人类基因组最强大的选择力量之一。特定疟疾相关基因的地理分布（撒哈拉以南非洲的达菲抗原和镰状细胞，地中海沿岸的地中海贫血和G6PD缺乏症）提供了有关疟疾历史分布的证据。然而，由于预防疟疾的基因所带来的副作用只是影响人类健康的众多因素之一，因此，人类遗传学和病原体基因所传达的信息有时很复杂。例如，在传统上，研究者认为，撒哈拉以南非洲没有达菲抗原，表明其是间日疟原虫的起源地。对间日疟原虫基因组的研究使这个问题变得复杂起来，因为间日疟原虫与东南亚的猕猴（猴子）疟疾联系最紧密，这表明可能是间日疟原虫从亚洲进入非洲之后，或是在防止疟疾或其他类似疟疾的其他种类寄生虫时出现了达菲阴性。然而，最近在野生大猩猩粪便样本中发现的疟疾DNA再次使证据重新倾向于间日疟的非洲起源。

除了人类进化出的对抗疟疾的基本防御系统（无论是否感染过疟疾，这些系统都是存在的）之外，人类的适应性免疫系统也在预防疟疾中扮演了重要角色。不幸的是，与麻疹等简单的急性病毒性疾病所诱发的快速且基本上终身免疫反应不同，疟疾引发的免疫反应发展较慢。没有人完全知晓其中的原因，尽管不同种类的疟原虫之间的分子标记存在巨大差异，而且单个疟疾克隆能够改变其分子外观，但人们认为这只是原因之一。在疟疾高发地区，人们通常在儿童时期就对疟疾产生了耐受性，

72

因为他们已经感染过几次疟疾。疟疾免疫力通常会很快消失，部分原因可能是疟原虫干扰了人体免疫系统。

另一个问题是，人类对抗疟疾所产生的适应性免疫提供了更多的耐受性（也被称为**临床免疫力**），而不是抵抗力。换言之，免疫确实减少了血液中疟原虫的数量，但其主要作用是减轻症状的严重程度。这种耐受性有两个重要的意义：（1）在疟疾高发区，具有临床免疫力的人感染疟疾后可能也不会出现明显的症状，故即使有治疗方法，他们也不会得到治疗，这就更难降低疟疾的高发病率；（2）当疟疾发病率和临床免疫力水平降低时，控制疟疾发病率就相对更容易。

在历史进程的大部分时间里，大多数人都是避开疟疾高发地区（如果可以选择的话）或与疟疾共存，希望通过自然免疫力在一定程度上减轻临床症状来对抗疟疾。我们对疟疾的历史认识，始于人类首次尝试有意识地去抵御疟疾。早在发现疟疾病原体之前，人类就发现了阻断疟疾相容筛选的化学防御措施。17世纪初，耶稣会士将从树皮中提取的传统药物奎宁带入欧洲。因为南美原住民咀嚼金鸡纳树的树皮可以止抖，耶稣会士猜测，它可能对疟疾引起的发热有效，因为疟疾所致的发热往往伴随着寒战。耶稣会士们很幸运；奎宁实际上并不能退烧，但确实能治愈疟疾，因为它能使疟原虫在血液寄生阶段所产生的有毒化学物质积聚起来。

73

虽然奎宁可以治疗疟疾，但价格昂贵，毒性太大，不适宜作为普遍疗法。如有可能，通过关闭相遇筛选阻止传播，比在发生传播后关闭相容筛选来预防疟疾花费更少且更安全。这种策略适用于许多疾病。不需要科技含量的解决方案，如一夫一妻制，戴避孕套，使用干净的针头，洗手时用洗手液或特殊的盛水容器，比效果最好的疫苗和治疗方法都更有效（如果你能让人们使用它们）。

对于消灭疟疾而言，综上可以得出结论：控制疟疾的传播（例如，通过覆盖水容器以消除幼蚊的适宜栖息地）可能比治疗疟疾感染者更有效。有时候，蚊子数量减少，疟疾由此得以控制，是作为土地利用变化的副作用自然发生的；农业实践的变化则减少了可用于蚊虫繁殖的积水量，人们认为，这是19世纪末美国北部疟疾减少的原因。当然，土地利用的改变可以在这两个方面发挥作用。20世纪30年代，美国南部农田的废弃增加了疟疾感染率。最近，肯尼亚西部的疟疾发病率，随着活跃的制砖坑数量的增加而增加，这些制砖坑可以蓄水，但往往很少有食蚊的天敌，为蚊子幼虫提供了完美的栖息地。

在发现滴滴涕之前，公共卫生部门会与工程师合作，通过管理水源来减少蚊子幼虫的栖息地，如排干沼泽里的水或增加水流量或改变水位，使当地传播疟疾的蚊虫无处栖息。他们还在水中喷洒油类或砷类杀虫剂来杀灭幼虫。在生物防治方面，卫生部门引进了食幼虫的鱼类，特别是**食蚊鱼属**，因其饮食习惯而被称为食蚊鱼。20世纪上半叶，食蚊鱼从北美被引进到世界各地的疟疾地区，从南美到中亚，从意大利到巴勒斯坦。然而，很难确切知道食蚊鱼防控疟疾的效果究竟如何，因为生物防治通常与其他控制措施，如水源管理和化学喷雾等相结合。

虽然这种减源形式在发达国家、温带或半干旱地区以及疟疾传播缓慢的地区有一定成效，但对于疟疾猖獗的贫穷国家及潮湿的热带地区来说，这种方式往往不切实际。1939年，保罗·赫尔曼·穆勒发现了滴滴涕的杀虫特性，并因此获得了1948年的诺贝尔奖，这一发现使疟疾的防控发生了革命性的变化。它引发了一场环境和生态工程的转变，从致力于消灭栖息地中的蚊类幼虫，转变为通过消灭人类附近的成年蚊子进行预防。室内残留喷洒方案将长效杀虫剂涂抹在蚊子喜欢落脚的房屋表面。如果有廉价、长效、对人体无害的杀虫剂（如滴滴涕），这种方案效果非常好。根据气候和墙面的特点，房屋可能每年仅需喷涂几次。一般来说，残留喷洒比驱赶蚊子的效果更好——不仅因为价格便宜，而且还能杀死蚊子，故可在房屋周围地区提供一些保护。残留喷洒方案在世界各地取得了初步成功：经过数十年努力，疟疾源头得到有效控制，美国终于在20世纪50年代初消灭了疟疾，而许多非洲国家的残留喷洒方案（使用滴滴涕和其他杀虫剂），至少在初期很大程度上降低了疟疾的疾病负担。

75

第二次世界大战后，在疟疾防治方面的第二个重大进展是氯喹的研发，氯喹是一种与奎宁相似的抗疟药，但价格更便宜且毒性更小。氯喹是第一次世界大战后由德国科学家首次合成的，当时盟军控制了爪哇岛，而爪哇岛拥有全球大部分的奎宁原材料，使得东非德军失去了这类重要药物。在第二次世界大战期间，当日本人占领爪哇岛时，情况发生了转变；美国的研究人员随后将氯喹开发成一种有效的抗疟药，虽然为时已晚而无法救治他们的士兵（那时士兵们位于西西里岛和东南亚）。大规模使用氯喹既可以治疗疟疾患者，改善个人健康，又可以减少疟疾患者将病原体传染给蚊子的机会，从而降低了疟疾在人群中的威胁。除上述优点外，氯喹还有助于控制大多数疟原虫的性阶段，从而阻断传播，并治疗感染者。

滴滴涕和氯喹以及其他合成杀虫剂和治疗方法的综合效力，使全球卫生机构在20世纪50年代非常乐观地认为疟疾可以得到控制，甚至可以根除。然而，在抗药性最强的地区——贫穷及热带国家的农村地区，疟疾的防治工作在几十年后遇到了意想不到的问题。尽管滴滴涕和氯喹相对便宜、无毒和有效，但开展全球疟疾防治运动的财政和后勤困难比任何人想象的都要大。

76

首先，与所有帮助欠发达国家人民的运动一样，疟疾防控方案也遇到了后勤、行政和文化方面的障碍。当地政府是否真的将物资送到最需要的地方？人们是否会擅自将这些物资用作其他用途？交通是否便利，可以把物资送达吗？如果物资到达目的地，是否能培训人们正确使用？当地居民可能不想使用滴滴涕，因为它的气味很难闻，而且会弄脏墙壁。他们可能会反感外来入侵，因而可能会爆发冲突，并中断防控计划，一切都回到原点。慈善机构可能在几年后就厌倦了捐款，或者他们可能会决定解决其他更重要的问题，如为受饥群众提供食物，或者提供清洁的水源，或者预防埃博拉等其他疾病。

全球疟疾根除计划始于1955年，目标是在1963年之前消灭疟疾，虽然该计划确实将疟疾的死亡率从1900年的基线降低了十倍以上，但在1969年最终放弃该计划之前，它遇到了上述所有的问题，甚至更多。这项运动的另一个意想不到的问题是，蕾切尔·卡森在1962年出版的《寂静的春天》中宣传了滴滴涕的使用与北美鸟类死亡的联系，导致滴滴涕在美国及加拿大先后被禁止使用。

其次，与所有传染病的防控工作一样，我们交战的敌人是生物体，它们会针对控制策略演变出相应的对策。疟疾病媒（对抗滴滴涕和其他合成杀虫剂）和病原体本身（对抗氯喹和其他合成抗疟疾药物）均会产生抗药性。化学防控的基本原则是毒害目标生物体——引入一种破坏其生理或生化等方面的化学物质，而不会对宿主（因为化学治疗药剂）或自然环境中的其他物种（因为病媒控制剂）造成太大的毒性。然后，目标生物体会处于自然选择的强大压力之中，要么改变其生物学特性，以中和化学物质的影响，要么研发出解毒化学物质或从其细胞中去除化学物质的方法。

77

蚊子通过遗传突变将这种化学物质排出细胞，从而获得对氯喹的抵抗力。没有人知道这些突变最初发生的确切时间，但它们传播速度很快；恶性疟原虫对氯喹的抗药性最早是在20世纪50年代末在南美和东南亚发现的，并于20世纪70年代在非洲出现。到了2005年左右，氯喹抗药性已经在全球蔓延。幸运的是，中国研究人员在筛选历史上已用于治疗发热的药物时，重新发现了一种名为青蒿素的新型抗疟药。青蒿素现已成为疟疾治疗的一线首选药物；然而，目前在东南亚地区，青蒿素也已经进化出部分抗药性。世界卫生组织正在积极努力地防止抗药性蔓延，主要是确保青蒿素要始终与其他抗疟疾药物联合使用，从根本上降低疟原虫同时对两种药物产生抗药性的可能性，这与HAART方案治疗HIV时，HIV产生抗药性类似，因为会同时使用三种药物，故上述情况极少出现。

对滴滴涕具有抗药性的蚊子具有遗传修饰，可改变其神经元（滴滴涕的靶点）的生化特性，或使神经元在体内分解滴滴涕。20世纪50年代中期已经发现蚊子对滴滴涕产生了抗药性，如今已经很普遍，不过不同种类及不同国家的蚊子，抗药性水平差异很大。一些研究人员认为，对滴滴涕的抗药性在很大程度上与其在农业上的大量使用有关（主要针对其他昆虫，但蚊子同时也暴露在滴滴涕中），如果滴滴涕仅用于传染病的防控，其效果可能更佳。虽然原则上，如果某一地区停止使用滴滴涕，蚊子也会失去对滴滴涕的抗药性，但在苍蝇身上的实验表明，对滴滴涕的抗药性程度较轻，就算有，似乎也没有适应成本，因此，蚊子对滴滴涕的抗药性可能会持续很长时间。疟疾防控方案现在试图通过轮流使用各种不同的合成杀虫剂来管理抗药性，这些合成杀虫剂的成本、对蚊子的效力，以及对人类或其他昆虫或野生动物的毒性各不相同。

在过去几十年中，国际社会再次加大了根除和控制疟疾的力度。策略制定者从早期方案的失败中吸取了教训：尤其是他们更加意识到政治和文化背景的重要性，在不同地区使用不同防控策略的重要性，并将疟疾控制方案视为全面改善卫生基础设施一部分的重要性。他们还降低了对根除疟疾的乐观态度：新的国际计划被称为全球疟疾**行动**（而不是“根除”）计划（GMAP），其目标只是从特定国家当地消除疟疾。虽然GMAP的确指出，随着疟疾在部分国家被消除，用于疟疾防控的支出可能会减少，因此，只需要资金来维持疟疾的消灭状态。目前的支出率约为每年25亿美元，而控制和根除疟疾可能需要80亿至100亿美元，这种水平的防控开支可能需要维持几十年。

如今，有了一种在20世纪60年代尚未出现的新型预防疟疾的工具——使用拟除虫菊酯的驱虫蚊帐，拟除虫菊酯是一种对哺乳动物安全的杀虫剂（但对鱼类有毒）。这种驱虫蚊帐最早是在20世纪80年代纳入了部署；21世纪初长效型驱虫蚊帐问世，其灭蚊的效果可保持五年，比最初有效期为六个月的驱虫蚊帐更有效。拟除虫菊酯驱虫蚊帐的概念与室内残留喷洒相似——都能杀死室内叮咬人的蚊子，但驱虫蚊帐有额外的优势，即同时提供物理和化学屏障，甚至在有多孔墙壁而不适合喷洒的房屋中也能发挥作用。蚊帐有其后勤和文化方面的问题，例如，据了解，受援者用蚊帐来捕鱼或晾晒鱼，而不是用来预防疟疾。然而，鉴于没有任何一项疟疾控制策略是百分之百有效的，因此驱虫蚊帐是对疟疾防控策略的重要补充。

79

蚊帐的一个教训是，与短效的工具相比，长效工具几乎总是更好的——更具成本效益，且花费精力更少。在其他条件不变的情况下，每五年更换一次的蚊帐要比每六个月重复一次的残留喷洒计划更好，虽然蚊帐只有在人们睡在里面时才起作用。疟疾疫苗，即使是一种不完美且短效的疫苗，也将是蚊帐的相容筛选类似物。与其在感染后才用青蒿素治疗，不如每隔几年就接种一次疫苗。目前（截至2015年1月）尚无可用的疟疾疫苗，但最有希望的疫苗已计划在未来几年内使用，该疫苗的临床试验结果表明，对儿童的保护率有25%—50%。研究人员认为，在某些地区，疫苗比蚊帐更具成本效益。

我们仍然对疟原虫所知甚少。进一步了解各类疟原虫在何时何地进入人类种群的古老历史，将加深我们对产生新型人类菌株的人畜共患过程的理解。同时了解疟疾在非人灵长类动物中的分布和生态，可以帮助我们预估未来人畜共患病发生的可能性。增加对野生种群的采样，以及对疟疾和灵长类基因组进行更快、更便宜的基因组扫描，有助于解决这一问题，但谁也不 80 知道我们能在多大程度上完全了解疟疾的生态学或进化史。

那么，疟疾防治的未来会怎样呢？我们可以持乐观态度。如果发展中国家没有受到重大的经济或政治冲击，或者没有新发或再发使人们不再关注疟疾的病原体，那么许多国家和基金会目前的努力将在今后几十年中继续减轻疟疾的疾病负担。在许多地区消灭疟疾是可能的，但疟疾专家对消灭疟疾的前景充其量只是持谨慎乐观的态度。

与蚊子和疟疾的进化同步，气候变化以及（更重要的）土地利用和经济变化将不断推动这一目标的实现。没有灵丹妙药能解决疟疾问题。各国政府和机构必须采取适合当地情况的措施，将现有防控手段（源头控制、残留喷洒、蚊帐、治疗以及最终 81 的疫苗）进行不同的组合来控制疟疾。

第七章

蛙壶菌

蛙壶菌是我们最后一个讨论的案例，它与上述疾病或病原体有许多不同之处。这种真菌是我们将讨论的第一种（也是唯一的）非人类病原体。它的基因组比前文介绍的病毒和细菌的基因组大很多倍，与疟原虫的基因组大小相似。蛙壶菌是一种分布广泛的病原体，能感染数百种不同的两栖动物，其中一些物种甚至因此灭绝。

最重要的是，蛙壶菌是我们所介绍的第一个**新发**病原体。实际上，新发病原体的定义非常广泛；它本质上是指我们由于某种原因而新近关注的病原体。这种病原体可能是真正通过突变而出现的新型病原体。更常见的是，当现有病原体传播给一个新物种时，人畜共患病原体就会出现。当我们在已知宿主体内检测到以前已知的病原体，但是在全新的地理环境中发现的，我们也可以将这类疾病归类为新发疾病。另外，新发也可以用来描述现有病原体的毒性或传播性的增加（由于突变，或由于宿主或自然环境的某些变化）。

最后，由于基因或环境的变化，宿主的耐受性或抵抗力可能会降低。

对于人类的新发病原体，主要是指人畜共患病（如艾滋病），82 有时还与病原体突变（如大流行性流感）相结合。当环境变化打开了现有传染病的环境筛选时，人类病原体也会出现，例如当登革热的蚊媒传播到北美时，或者当人们在林区建房时，也增加了与引发莱姆病的蜱虫的接触。

非人类物种新发疾病引发人们的关注，主要有几点原因。许多非人类物种具有经济价值；新发疾病可能威胁我们的钱包，甚至我们的生命。农业疾病会威胁到重要的农作物。爱尔兰马铃薯枯萎病的病原体是真菌，其起源于南美，经由北美传播到欧洲，造成了大量感染者死亡，并从根本上改变了爱尔兰的历史。

疾病也会影响具有重要经济意义的野生种群。最近蜜蜂数量减少，其原因仍在激烈争论中，但部分原因是病原体传播，严重影响了靠蜜蜂授粉的加利福尼亚杏仁作物；野生麋鹿的慢性消耗病有可能使加拿大麋鹿养殖者损失数百万美元。我们也希望出于无私的原因关心非人类生物的福祉——保护非人类物种只是在做正确的事。

两栖动物中的蛙壶菌肯定属于后一类——尽管一些两栖类物种在蛙腿贸易或消灭害虫方面具有经济价值，但大多数受蛙壶菌影响的物种并没有太大的经济价值。然而，我们想了解蛙壶菌的来源，并探索该如何保护野生两栖动物种群免受蛙壶菌的影响。在确定蛙壶菌来源时使用的概念和策略，也可以作为 83 了解和控制未来出现的非人类物种疾病的案例研究。

生理学和自然史

壶菌是一类大型真菌家族，但大多鲜为人知，蛙壶菌则是壶菌中的异类。虽然有少数蛙壶菌攻击其他真菌或植物，但大多数都以水生环境中腐烂的有机物为食，对人体无害。蛙壶菌是已知的且仅有的两种攻击脊椎动物的壶菌之一，第二种是2013年才发现的一种蝾螈壶菌。（当人们将蛙壶菌称为“壶菌”时，壶菌类生物学家抱怨道，这种叫法不公平，会让所有壶菌类的名声都被其中一个物种的不端行为所玷污。）蛙壶菌生活在两栖动物的皮肤上和皮下，特别是在角蛋白上，这是一种在皮肤中发现的硬蛋白质。它的生命周期在被称为**菌体**的结构和**游动孢子**之间交替。菌体是生长在宿主皮肤层内的瓶状细胞，游动孢子是由菌体散布到水中的小型移动细胞，最终落回同一个宿主的皮肤上，或是落在另一个宿主身上，从而传播感染。

我们对蛙壶菌何时及如何在远离宿主机体的自然环境中持续存在知之甚少。如果我们想了解蛙壶菌如何从一个两栖动物种群传播到另一个种群；若某一种群在当地被蛙壶菌灭绝后是否能恢复或重新定殖；以及如何设计隔离方案来保护健康群体免受蛙壶菌的影响至关重要。鉴于蛙壶菌的许多亲属都是自由生活的微生物，如果蛙壶菌也保留了在自然环境中生存和生长的能力也就不足为奇了。我们知道，蛙壶菌可以在纯净的水中持续生存数周或数月，并在两栖动物的皮肤、羽毛以及昆虫和甲壳类动物（如虾和小龙虾）的外骨骼中的角蛋白上生长。然而，目前我们还不知道它们是否能在没有宿主的情况下生存数年，或者进行远距离的传播。

蛙壶菌可能在季节交替时在蝌蚪身上存活。这一生命阶84段的耐受性较强，因为蝌蚪的嘴周围只有角质，它们可能会在受到感染的情况下丢弃这些角质但不会死亡。这种形式的**种内储存**，即病原体在同一物种耐受性较好的生命阶段中持续存在，也在其他两栖动物的病原体中存在。许多种类的蝌蚪生长较慢，但感染蛙壶菌后不会死亡；但也有其他种类的蝌蚪确实因感染蛙壶菌而死亡。蛙壶菌感染最重要的储存库和载体可能是来自耐受性宿主物种，这些宿主可以窝藏真菌，并将其传给新的（或恢复中的）种群，且不会对自身造成伤害。大多数两栖动物群落都存在有耐受性的宿主——研究人员仍在探索是什么使宿主对蛙壶菌耐受或不耐受。部分最重要的潜在参与者是一些种类的小龙虾、美国牛蛙和南非的**非洲爪蟾**。这些物种分布广泛，无论是否有人类的帮助，都可以入侵新地区，并且对某些蛙壶菌菌株耐受。

我们不知道的另一个关于蛙壶菌的问题就是，它是如何杀死宿主的。研究人员推测了各种原因，包括蛙壶菌能产生某种致死性毒素。然而，目前的大部分证据表明，被感染的成年蛙，皮肤中聚积着大量蛙壶菌，随后皮肤会增厚和硬化，使蛙无法维持体内适当的盐浓度，从而导致心脏骤停而死亡。

两栖动物对蛙壶菌的易感性差异很大：在空间、时间、物种和群落上的巨大差异是这种新型传染病的特征。有些变异可能源于宿主防御的差异。非洲爪蟾的免疫系统能产生识别蛙壶菌的抗体，尽管目前只有微弱的证据表明，这些蛋白质能保护机体，抵抗真菌的侵害。然而，很多种类的青蛙和蟾蜍分泌的抗菌85肽，对皮肤有保护作用的证据更为有力；它们的皮肤分泌物在试管中能抑制蛙壶菌，也更容易在感染后存活下来。

最后，某些物种似乎有能力对蛙壶菌产生行为上的“发热”，蛙壶菌在十七至二十三摄氏度之间生长最快，但在三十摄氏度以上的温度下就会死亡。虽然青蛙是冷血动物，无法实现颤抖性产热，但被蛙壶菌感染的青蛙可以且确实会通过在温暖、阳光充足的地方多待一段时间来提高体温，这有助于它们康复。在实验室里，将感染的青蛙放在温暖的环境中不到一天，就可以治愈。并非所有物种都可以通过这种方式治愈，这表明高温不是直接损害蛙壶菌，而是可以通过提高青蛙产生抗菌肽的能力来抗感染。不同的研究人员，在不同的实验室，进行不同的实验程序，对不同的物种进行研究，也可以解释物种间存在的一些差异。

发 现

生态学家在20世纪90年代末发现了蛙壶菌，当时整个澳大利亚东部和中美洲的青蛙开始死于某个神秘的原因。与此同时，美国国家动物园的毒镖蛙也开始死亡。兽医科学家联系了世界上为数不多对这类鲜为人知的真菌家族有所了解的研究者。他们根据毒镖蛙的拉丁文名称提出了对这一物种的描述和名称：蛙壶菌，意思是“感染青蛙和蟾蜍的壶菌”。

蛙壶菌发现过程中有一个有趣的小插曲，是壶菌专家乔伊斯·朗科尔的经历。在家育儿二十年后，朗科尔重返研究生院，于1991年获得真菌学博士学位。1997年，就在蛙壶菌发现之前，她似乎已经准备好潜心研究一个不为人知的真菌家族。当蛙壶菌的重要性激增时，她成为了解壶菌生物学信息的关键人

86

物，她的事业也得以迅速发展。自1998年以来，她与人合著了64篇论文，被引总数超过3 700次，成了科研明星。她的故事证明了在关键时刻掌握正确知识的价值。这也说明，看似玄奥的生物学知识，在理解一种新的生态环境时，会变得至关重要。

在明确了蛙壶菌是一种新型病原体后，生物学家就开始探索它的起源：蛙壶菌是近年来才入侵其所破坏的种群的，还是已经在这些物种身上蛰伏了几千年才开始造成危害的？**新型病原体假说**（NPH）和地方流行**病原体假说**（EPH）自发现蛙壶菌起，就引发了激烈的争论，这两种假说适用于大多数新发的野生动物疾病。虽然在蛙壶菌被发现后的二十年里，我们已经掌握了大量关于蛙壶菌及其与两栖动物相互作用的信息，但争论仍在继续：每次一项新的研究支持NPH，另一项研究都会迅速跟进，为EPH添加证据。

NPH尚未指出蛙壶菌是一个新物种，我们知道它在20世纪90年代之前就早已经存在了。相反，该假说指出，对于目前受感染人群所在的特定地区来说，蛙壶菌或蛙壶菌的毒株是新物种。如果NPH是合理的，那么蛙壶菌一定是在首次发现与壶菌病有关的死亡时就入侵了新环境。根据该假说，在蛙壶菌已经入侵和还尚未入侵的区域之间应该有清晰的空间分隔，而不是在出现死亡和无死亡病例的地区有重合。我们还应该能够在蛙壶菌的基因空间分布中观察到它迅速传播的特征，在其长期存在的地区具有高度遗传多样性，而在最近暴发壶菌病的地区，遗传多样性较低。

87

与此相反，EPH称，在两栖动物群落中，甚至在最近暴发过疾病的群落中，相同的蛙壶菌菌株已经存在了很长时间。植物流行病学中的疾病三角理论认为，疾病暴发需要（1）合适的宿主，（2）病原体，（3）环境，病原体在其中可以克服相遇和相容筛选而发生传播，并能克服耐受性而引发疾病。EPH认为，“三角形”的“前两条边”已经存在了数百年或数千年，但最近自然环境的一些变化，打开了相遇和相容筛选，或改变了耐受性。由于蛙壶菌必须（据我们目前所知）感染两栖类宿主才能长期生存，所以不是相遇（传播）或相容（抵抗）筛选打开了；相反，EPH的支持者认为，自然环境的变化让宿主对蛙壶菌的耐受性降低，或者在同等情况下，使蛙壶菌的毒性变强。为了验证该假说，我们不仅要推翻NPH（蛙壶菌的空间分布及其遗传变异的空间模式应该充满了争议并且无法预测），还应该能够确定环境协变量，以预测宿主在特定群落中是否具有耐受/蛙壶菌是否具有毒性，并找到这些协变量最近在壶菌病暴发地区发生变化的证据。

在仔细研究每种假设的证据之前，需要牢记的是，如同所有的生物学现象一样，蛙壶菌的起源很复杂，而且上述两种假说并非是互斥的。蛙壶菌近年来已经传播到了新地区（如NPH所述），也可能是蛙壶菌毒力增强，或者宿主失去了耐受性（如EPH所述）。

我们先从历史和遗传证据开始分析，这些证据应该有助于确定蛙壶菌开始在全球范围内传播的时间。与所有动物性传染病一样，生物学家在两栖动物群落中发现蛙壶菌之前，就已经存在了。然而，与疟疾或流感等人类传染病不同的是，没有任何历史记录可以告诉我们，蛙壶菌在什么地方出现过——在古代，即使发生过青蛙和蟾蜍大量死亡的瘟疫，人们可能也不

88

会注意到。事实上，就算近代有关于两栖动物死亡的记载，比如20世纪70年代科罗拉多州山区北方蟾蜍的灭绝，或者20世纪80年代末中美洲**阿特洛普蛙**的减少，虽然我们回溯性地将两栖类动物死亡的原因归咎于蛙壶菌的入侵，但那时，人们却认为是其他原因，比如气候变化或环境压力加上细菌暴发，导致了这些物种的灭绝。

随着DNA鉴定法的出现，其类似于在埃及木乃伊中发现疟疾时运用的方法，科学家们能够检测收藏在自然历史博物馆中的蛙皮上的蛙壶菌DNA来追溯传播时间。在科罗拉多州和中美洲，研究者成功地从疫情暴发前后收集的青蛙皮中复原了蛙壶菌，这一进展让蛙壶菌导致两栖类动物死亡的推测变得合情合理。然而，这些结果并不能有力支持NPH和EPH，因为研究人员还不能证明这些地区在暴发前的一段时间内没有遭受过蛙壶菌的侵袭。

研究者们欣喜地发现，1938年在南非采集的非洲爪蟾的皮肤上能检测到蛙壶菌DNA。蛙壶菌的早期出现与非洲爪蟾这种分布广泛、耐受力强的物种有关，因此，研究者们提出“走出非洲”假说，即后来引发全球蛙壶菌大流行的菌株早在1938年以前，就开始在非洲进化，直到20世纪30年代，随着基于非洲爪蟾卵的人类妊娠试验开展，每年从南非出口成千上万只非洲爪蟾，蛙壶菌才开始在全球蔓延。根据该假设，在20世纪40年代和50年代（在其他妊娠试验取代非洲爪蟾卵试验之前），这种真菌将有二十年的时间在全球传播，此后，蛙壶菌可能通过其他耐受性宿主逐渐在新的环境传播。

然而，这些假设不堪一击，每当有科学家从年代更久远的

89

两栖动物皮肤上发现了蛙壶菌，并创造了新纪录时，情况就发生了变化。2013年和2014年的两项发现彻底改变了争论的理由。首先，研究人员在1928年从加利福尼亚州采集的牛蛙皮肤上发现了蛙壶菌。牛蛙先前被怀疑在两栖动物群落中传播蛙壶菌。这一发现并没有完全排除“走出非洲”的假说，但它使该假设极大地复杂化了。由于在加利福尼亚发现的蛙壶菌，对非洲爪蟾的妊娠试验驱动爪蟾出口来说还为时过早，要证实这一假说，蛙壶菌必须在十年前通过其他方法传播出非洲，或是在加利福尼亚州的蛙皮中发现的菌株必须与非洲爪蟾是不同（非病毒性）的族系。随后，一组研究人员有了更轰动的发现，其在巴西大西洋森林中四分之一的青蛙身上发现了蛙壶菌，这些青蛙都是从1894年开始收集的。

虽然研究人员会不断推翻这些纪录，在全球范围内发现蛙壶菌更早期的踪迹，但随着时间的推移，新的发现会越来越艰难，因为博物馆中能检测的蛙皮标本越来越少。而从蛙壶菌基因组的证据来看，我们再次发现蛙壶菌的很多方面都很复杂。蛙壶菌有很多族系，其中最重要的（从我们的观点来看）是**全球大流行谱系**（GPL），它记录了所有从数量呈下降趋势的两栖动物种群中收集到的样本和一些其他的样本。在对蛙壶菌进行首次系统发育的研究中，GPL有传播速度快的病原体家族的确切特征：其成员之间的遗传变异水平非常低，并且缺乏可识别的地理模式，这些都可以用病原体定居新群落的速度远远快于在特定地区进化出特有新基因型的过程来解释。最近的研究再次使情况复杂化。虽然GPL在地理上仍然很混乱，涵盖了来自每个地区的代表性蛙壶菌菌株，但不断增长的数据库和逐步完善的

90

基因组扫描表明，该谱系也包含了高度变异的病原体；最新的研究已经将GPL中祖先的估计年龄从短短几十年（与一种新出现的病原体一致，该病原体最初起源于非洲爪蟾出口时期）到至少一万年。此外，来自巴西青蛙的直接历史证据表明，无论该谱系起源自哪里，来自该谱系的蛙壶菌菌株实际上在南美洲已经存在了一个世纪，显然该菌株未导致两栖动物群落的种群减少和灭绝。

我们希望可以对博物馆收藏的蛙皮进行更多的分析及更全面的基因组扫描，或许还能厘清目前被定名为GPL的各类谱系的历史。更深入的研究最终可能成功地将GPL在世界各地存在了数千年的菌株，全部分为低毒力组和新的、可能是由现有菌株杂交产生的高毒力组。数十年来随着蛙壶菌从一个地区扩散到另一个地区，新高毒力组已导致20世纪70年代科罗拉多州、80年代中美洲，以及21世纪前十年澳大利亚东部和中美洲蛙壶菌感染的两栖动物数量下降。

另一方面，数据未能提供令人信服的、简单的证据来支持NPH，这可能会导致研究人员将重心重新转移到EPH。在早期，即在中美洲和澳大利亚的下降之后，尤其是当蛙壶菌对两栖类动物的影响在种群之间发生明显变化时，研究人员争先恐后地寻找环境变化，以解释蛙壶菌毒力（明显地）突然改变。有一个令人费解的问题是，致命性蛙壶菌似乎经常出现在自然保护区等海拔较高的原始地区，与人为改变环境的故事相矛盾。科学家们最初认为，有两个环境因素，即农药污染（可能是从农业地区远距离带来的）和紫外线辐射（与海拔影响结果一致），可能与蛙壶菌相互作用，通过给两栖动物加压或抑制其

91

免疫反应而致死。尽管与种群数量下降有关，而且一些实验室研究表明，紫外线辐射和杀虫剂可以增加蛙壶菌的毒性，但这些因素（目前）尚不能为预测蛙壶菌何时何地攻击两栖动物群落提供很大的帮助。

温度具有更强的信号：温度与蛙壶菌对实验室研究中动物个体和自然界中种群产生的有害影响有关。如上所述，研究表明，蛙壶菌的适宜温度窗口很窄，其生存环境的温度在窗口内时，毒力最强。温度有可能解释高海拔地区两栖类动物的灭亡模式，因为高海拔地区的温度一直较低。然而，虽然它可以解释为什么低洼地区的群落持续存在，而其生活在高海拔地区的邻居却被疾病摧毁，但它不能解释时间模式——如果蛙壶菌已经存在了几个世纪，为什么高海拔群落只是在过去几十年才开始被摧毁，而之前从未发生？到底发生了什么变化？

最明显的可能因素——也是环保主义者一直关注的问题——就是人类活动引起的气候变化。我们知道气候变化会严重影响高纬度和高海拔地区的生态群落，或许近年来的气候变化已经改变了气候条件，使其超过了一个临界点，通过提高蛙壶菌的生长速度（例如，游动孢子的繁殖速度）或降低两栖动物的相容筛选，从而使蛙壶菌扩散和/或危害群落。

92

气候变化假说在蛙壶菌研究界一直存在争议。2006年，一项备受瞩目的研究表明，中美洲高原日温温差变化的减少，可以使蛙壶菌在其最佳温度范围内保持更长时间，从而促进了蛙壶菌的暴发。其他科学家指出，这项研究在一些重要的细节上有纰漏，如温度变化、蛙壶菌暴发和种群灭亡时间的滞后。此外，两栖类动物灭亡的空间模式——以每年数百公里的速度在中美洲蔓延，而不是同时影响整个地区——似乎更符合新型病原体传播的特征，而不是区域气候的变化。为了验证最初的假设，随后使用相同的气候和死亡数据以及额外的气候测量数据进行的分析表明，即使考虑到传播的空间模式，温度变异性的变化而非平均温度的变化确实与物种灭绝有关，而物种灭绝可能是由被称为厄尔尼诺的全球十年尺度气候变化的局部效应造成的，而不是受人类活动引起的气候变化的影响。一项关于蛙壶菌灭亡的全球性研究发现，年降水量与灭亡相关，尽管其他类似研究未能发现明显的影响。虽然气候的变化很可能是导致蛙壶菌暴发及其影响的原因，但它们并没有提供EPH支持者正在寻找的确凿证据。

随着蛙壶菌的故事逐渐变得复杂，许多生物学家承认，无论是NPH还是EPH都不能说明全部问题。我们是否需要进一步探究蛙壶菌的起源时间、地点和原因，以及它对两栖动物种群造成的严重后果？虽然科学有时好像在兜圈子——研究人员仍然专注于最初发现蛙壶菌时引发争论的假说；但进一步的研究指出，令人欣慰的是，蛙壶菌的研究之路更像一个不断缩小的螺旋线。虽然再度回到相同的论点，但这次是以新的复杂程度，并掌握了新的证据，并站在了更高的层次上。从近年及以前采集到的蛙皮中提取的蛙壶菌基因组数据，让我们对这类壶菌在空间和时间上的分布有了更深入的了解，几种新技术的运用有望给我们提供更多的信息。来自两栖动物宿主的基因组数据，可以提供过去关于种群研究瓶颈的证据；观察抗菌蛋白的基因可以提示过去哪些物种需要抵御蛙壶菌。在EPH方面，曾经关于气候的代指物，如树木或土壤的同位素组成（揭示了温度和干燥的

93

模式），可以让我们更完整地了解宿主—病原体—环境疾病的三角关系在古老环境中的相互作用方式。

除了知识上的满足，这些信息是否有助于我们控制蛙壶菌的暴发或减少其对两栖动物群落的影响？NPH和EPH的争论对蛙壶菌的防控策略有一定的影响。如果NPH是正确的，这意味着自然环境**并没有**发生重要的变化，新出现的是病原体的存在，那么保护者应该把重点放在防止跨群落传播上。如果EPH是正确的，即病原体一直存在，但自然环境恶化了，那么我们应该担心如何让两栖动物的自然环境变得更好，以便它们能够抵抗或耐受蛙壶菌。

然而，这两种方法在实际生活中的作用可能没有早期看起来那么大。**如果**我们能够进行干预，逆转病原体的存在或自然环境的变化，那么我们就能保护两栖动物。但是，一旦蛙壶菌到达自然环境中，要将其从自然环境中移除是不现实的，我们无法改变厄尔尼诺事件或人类活动导致全球变化的发生（至少在有效的时间跨度上不能）。保护措施必须建立在我们认为能够从根本上解决疾病产生原因的基础上，这些行动是合乎道德规范的（为了拯救其他物种，是否可以宰杀一些濒危动物？），并在逻辑上是可行的。

94

即使对这种疾病一无所知，我们也可以通过将动物从野外转移到没有疾病的人工栖息地来关闭相遇筛选。“两栖动物方舟”是一个旨在保护物种的项目，无论自然界发生什么变化，该项目都会确保在圈养繁殖计划中都有一些动物，只要我们找到了控制蛙壶菌的方法，这些动物就可以（有希望）重新回归野外。生物学家已经成功地人工饲养了濒危物种，但我们不知道什么时候或如何才能重新将其引入自然环境。人工饲养可以赢得时间，但最终我们或需要培育这些物种的抗蛙壶菌变种，或是需要找到一种方法来防护自然界中的蛙壶菌。这也引发了伦理问题，将动物从野外转移是否会损害濒危物种？圈养种群的存在是否会降低我们处理这一问题的紧迫性？是否可以通过出售更多的圈养动物来筹集保护资金？

与其他疾病的控制和预防方案一样，防治蛙壶菌面临着两个基本问题：缺乏理论知识和资源。无论受害动物有多可爱或有趣，野生动物的疾病永远不会像人类疾病一样引起人们的兴趣，对此，我们总是拥有更少的资源和知识，因为获取知识需要资源。我们也确实有一些优势，如果有助于控制疾病暴发，我们可以扑杀动物、培育动物的疾病耐受性或抵抗力，并诱导实验性感染来评估治疗（从人类病原体控制的角度，这些策略均无益处）。由于尚未实地部署任何疾病控制策略，因此我们不必担心病原体采取的进化对策，虽然一旦开始采取防控，上述情况必然会发生。

虽然野生动物的传染病与人类的传染病在表面上有所不同，但驱动它们的生理、生态和进化动力学却非常相似。从长远来看，分析野生动物疾病有助于我们了解传染病的基本特征。它可以帮助保护具有经济价值的采伐或狩猎种群。了解疾病在自然种群中的传播方式可能还可以提供预警系统，以检测可能感染人类的人畜共患疾病。也许最根本的是，许多生物学家（包括本书的作者）认为，我们有道德责任在可能的情况下保护物种，特别是当人类活动可能导致威胁它们安全的疾病传播时。

第八章

展望未来

本书对一些重要的传染病及其生态和进化原理，以及这些原理如何为治疗和疾病控制提供依据进行了旋风式的考察。我们根据社会经济的重要性和生态/进化的兴趣，选择了一些可以纳入本书的案例研究，这些案例涵盖了广泛的致病类群。诚然，这些选择偏重于我们认为读者熟悉的疾病。

令人遗憾的是，我们仍遗漏了许多传染病，这些疾病夺去了数十万人的生命，降低了数百万伤残调整生命年，并且造成了数十亿美元的损失。比如结核病（被忽视的最重要的疾病）、小儿麻痹症和血吸虫病（一种造成肝脏损害的寄生虫病，主要对撒哈拉以南非洲的人群造成危害）。许多此类疾病在不发达的热带国家非常猖獗，以至于有了一个完整的类别——“被忽视的热带疾病”，并有一本科学杂志专门讨论这些疾病。

我们还遗漏了那些影响历史的致命性疾病。鼠疫，有史以来危害最大的传染病，号称传染病杀手，现在用抗生素治疗相对容易。天花，第一个在野外通过接种疫苗消灭的疾病，它摧毁了

97 美洲的土著居民，并被用来促进欧洲的殖民化。最后，与麻疹密切相关的牛病，即可能改变东非地貌的牛瘟，因为它灭绝了当地的野生动物，让灌木丛生的植被生长，促使舌蝇繁殖，并因此引起了一种叫昏睡病或锥虫病的媒传疾病。

在大多数情况下，我们关注的是已知疾病，而不是新发疾病，比如HIV和蛙壶菌是最近几年才出现的，2009年大流行的H1N1流感病毒也可以算作"最近出现的"。我们没有空间讨论新型冠状病毒，如SARS或MERS；鸡病毒，如尼帕病毒，其有可能从澳大利亚和东南亚的果蝠身上传播蔓延；或新发媒传疾病，如西尼罗河病毒和登革病毒，以及导致莱姆病的细菌。

最后，我们只介绍了一小部分可引起传染病的生物种类。不可否认，流感病毒和HIV等病毒、霍乱弧菌等细菌、恶性疟原虫等原生动物，以及蛙壶菌等真菌，构成了绝大多数的病原体。然而，我们还忽略了多细胞寄生虫，如蛔虫（线虫）和扁虫（扁形虫），传统意义上，它们被认为与微生物寄生虫传染病是分开的（见第二章），但与传染病病原体有着相同的流行病学、生态学和进化原理。多细胞寄生虫和原生动物引起了大部分被忽视的热带疾病。这些疾病一般只在相对贫穷的欠发达国家进行传播，而且它们通常导致慢性衰弱性疾病，而不是急性疾病，所以这类疾病在传统上被归为单独的类别。

在过去的几十年里，研究人员还发现了几种新型传染病模98 式，就像科幻小说一样。第一种是**朊病毒**，或叫可传播的感染性蛋白质，是一种错误折叠的蛋白质，它们可以通过催化其他蛋白质错误折叠成朊病毒的形式在宿主体内复制。朊病毒疾病，比如自1700年以来感染绵羊的羊瘙痒症，以及20世纪60年代在科罗拉多州被首次发现感染鹿的慢性消耗性疾病，这类疾病很可能是动物摄入了被朊病毒蛋白污染的植物后，在不同的动物群落中进行了传播。朊病毒蛋白通过被动物体液（唾液、粪便或羊水）污染的环境或从动物尸体释放到土壤中，进入植物体内，完成传播循环。

朊病毒疾病在20世纪90年代因"疯牛病"而引起人们的广泛关注，其正式名称为"牛海绵状脑病"（当这种病发生在人类身上时，则被称为"变异型克雅氏病"）。除了担心感染一种致命性神经系统退化的疾病之外，英国人对牛群中怪异行为，即无意识同类相食的暴发原因产生了浓厚的兴趣。为了促进它们的生长，这些动物被喂养了由牛大脑和脊髓组织组成的蛋白质补充剂。朊病毒病极少在动物身上自发发生，也几乎不会因为罕见的基因缺陷而产生；当感染朊病毒的动物尸体混入其他数百种动物的食物中时，就会导致灾难。从20世纪初开始，由于巴布亚新几内亚的先民有"停尸食人"（即在仪式上吃他们已故亲属）的习俗，这种涉及人而不是牛的同类相食行为，导致一场类似但更为可怕的朊病毒病开始流行；但在20世纪中期，在巴布亚新几内亚先民放弃"停尸食人"的习俗后再次消失。

那么未来几十年，传染病的防控前景如何？它可能对我们自身及家人的健康及社会福利产生哪些影响？它是来自已知疾病还是新发疾病？未来疾病的生态和进化将如何变化？

首先，我们要知道"越是变化的东西，越是保持不变"。尽管我们对疾病传播的理解，以及能够关闭相容筛选的疫苗和治疗方法的发展，已经彻底改变了传染病的管理方式，但推动疾病生态系统发展的基本过程仍然没有改变。人类已经取得了一些巨大的成功：我们已经彻底消灭了天花和牛瘟；并且有消灭小儿麻痹症和麻疹的可能性，虽然由于社会、政治和经济的原因，最后一步无比困难；虽说难以想象根除HIV，但我们已经研发出新的治疗方法，控制艾滋病感染者（至少是那些有机会获得优质医疗服务的人）的病情进展，让他们的预期寿命与正常人一样。

然而，我们也失去了一些疾病防控的根据地：结核病再次出现，并且与HIV一起出现；控制疟疾的最初几十年里的乐观以失败告终；莱姆病、西尼罗河病毒和H1N1流感等新发疾病在动物群体中持续蔓延。也许最可怕的失败是我们发现，治疗MRSA、疟疾及结核病的药物可能产生抗药性，以及抗生素也出现抗药性，因此我们不得不再次审视那些梦魇般无法治疗的传染病。

一个没有传染病的未来是不现实的。自生命诞生以来，生物就相互寄生，任何干预都无法改变这种生物现象。新疾病将通过现有疾病的突变或重组，以及动物种群的溢出效应而产生，现有疾病将通过不断进化来摆脱人类的控制。我们能够做的是将疾病的影响降到最低，同时疾病将永远与人类同在应了然于心。我们可以减缓或阻止流行病的发生，减少疾病造成的死亡和痛苦，但是我们永远无法完全征服疾病。

100

在过去五十年里，我们对传染病的认识发生了哪些变化？在此期间，我们的重心从群体层面的治疗转向了个体治疗。在这一进程中我们学到了，与对受感染的个体的治疗相比，群体层面的治疗在阻止传染病方面仍然具有价值。最大限度地减少疾病影响的方法是，先将其发病率降到最低。我们了解到，在预防疾病的过程中，群体层面和个体层面的防控策略有协同作用。群体免疫现象就是这样一个例子（见第二章）。

案例研究表明，引发传染病的病原体在不断演变。结核病卷土重来，部分原因是导致结核病的细菌已经进化出对抗生素的抗药性。HIV宿主从灵长类动物转变为人类后，为能够在人体内更好地生存，HIV发生了进化。但要记住的是，突变是随机发生的。相对无害的细菌与携带危险致病基因的细菌或病毒之间的相遇也是如此。由于这种内在的随机性，生存下来的生物越少，病原体毒性增强的可能性就越小。可以这样想：如果有二十种病毒，而这些病毒对抗病毒药物发生突变而产生抗药性的概率仅为百万分之一，那么其中一种病毒发生这种罕见突变的概率极低。但如果有十亿种病毒，发生突变实际上就无法避免。因此，有效的疫苗接种或隔离等群体层面的干预措施，能让传染病的病原体保持在较低水平，其进化成更危险的病原体的概率就会降低。还是那句话，一分的预防胜似十分的治疗。过去传染病防控失败的教训之一是，现代分子生物学的研究具有局限性。当人体已经产生了快速且有效的免疫反应时，疫苗的研制是最简单的。对于像艾滋病、疟疾或结核病这些利用进化技巧（如外形变化）来逃避免疫反应的疾病，我们可能永远无法研制出像能根除天花或显著降低麻疹和小儿麻痹症发病率那样廉价且有效的疫苗。

在了解到防控利器的局限性后，我们可以采用新的技术来帮助检测疾病病原体并开展治疗。鉴定病毒或检测细菌对抗生素的抗药性，在以前往往需要几天到几周的时间。例如，病毒分类需要细致的显微镜镜下检查或耗时的免疫学技术。抗药性检测需评估细菌在含有各种抗生素的平板培养基上生长的能力。如今，可以在几小时内通过对细菌和病毒的基因组测序来进行诊断和鉴定。而且，这些技术不再是实验室里熟练的技术人员的专利，现在已经有了适合在野外条件下对未经处理的样本（如唾液或血液）进行测序的技术，而且成本也在逐月下降。这种基因分型技术在细菌感染中可能有用，比如作为噬菌体治疗的一部分，该技术可用于筛选出合适的噬菌体种类以对抗它们。

我们吸取的另一个教训是改变人类行为的力量和局限性。我们可以在进入林区后小心防范蜱虫叮咬，不与陌生人发生体液交换，咳嗽时待在家里（或让孩子待在家），从而轻松关闭多种疾病的相遇筛选。然而，改变行为的实际成本和经济成本，通常意味着我们会不断地暴露自己和他人，甚至解决措施（表面上）看起来相对简单时，甚至会造成严重的后果（比如感染HIV）时。对于本书的读者来说，这是一个好消息，你可以通过很多简单的方法来预防疾病的感染，如果不幸被感染，也可以采取相应措施，停止疾病的传播。但整体来说，人类是顽固的生物，我们有许多相互矛盾的优先事项——赚钱，或仅仅是节省一点时间，这些事情往往会胜过那些能使自己或其他人免于感染的做法。

疾病防控的重点之一就是要制定出更好的措施，诚实而有效地让公众了解疾病的危害和掌握控制疾病的方法。有时个人和群体的利益是有冲突的。比如在生病时待在家里不上班，可能纯粹是个人出于自私的原因而做出的错误决定，因为这样虽然让同事受益，但会损失一天的工资，并削减老板对我们的好感。我们必须更合理地设计鼓励公民遵守公共卫生目标的政策，在不过度限制个人自由的情况下合理制定奖惩措施。

人类对自然环境造成的持续压力，是另一个已经发生了改变的事实。城市化和人口增长加快了人类感染新病原体的速度，这些病原体主要由动物携带。当我们迁入以前未曾居住过的地区，或者改变环境时，与动物及其携带的寄生虫的接触率就会增加。不仅是热带疾病存在这样的情况，温带疾病（如莱姆病）也可能发生。人类正在以多种方式改变环境，包括清洁水源、移居现代化城市、破坏热带森林等，不管这些行为是好是坏，都将改变流行病的地域分布。

流行病学家们正就历史上最大规模的无控制实验——化石燃料向大气中释放二氧化碳，以及随之而来的全球气候变化——对疾病流行可能造成的影响展开激烈辩论。一方面，毫无疑问，生态变化会导致流行病学变化，已经发现许多物种的分布范围会随着气候变化而改变，蚊子等昆虫病媒亦是如此。在东非高原等特定地区，气温上升确实会导致疟疾发病率的上升。但是，气候变化对区域的影响是复杂的，涉及变异性、季节性模式和水文循环以及总体温度的变化。再加上生态系统与区域气候相互作用的复杂性和不可预测性，科学家们指出："尽管我们可以肯定气候变化将对疾病产生某种影响，但很难确切地知道其影响是什么。"

蚊子是一个有意思的问题。乍一看，灭蚊至少可以消灭我们所知道的蚊媒传播疾病，特别是消灭传播破坏性疾病的蚊子。但事实上，最近有人认为，科学家们太过专注于研究疟疾的抗药性问题，以至于在对蚊子发起攻击时可能完全忽略了总体效应。灭蚊需要采取干预措施，比如排干湿地和/或使用会伤害其他物种的杀虫剂。当然，蚊子也会对杀虫剂产生抗药性，就像疟疾会对抗疟药产生抗药性一样。但更重要的一点是：对于传染病的思考不能停滞不前。对任何一种防控措施过度自信（抗疟药），或对传染病这种需从多方面考虑的问题中任何一部分过度关注（例如，仅仅关注寄生虫的抗药性），都会限制我们解决问题的能力。

人类的健康并不仅仅是战胜邪恶的寄生虫，无论是用灵丹妙药，还是日常防范，甚至是两者兼而有之。寄生虫与我们一样，都是生活在同一个自然系统中。虽然本书中没有对这方面进行大篇幅叙述，但人类社会学对传染病的传播也有巨大的影响。在《圣经新约》中，"天启四骑士"分别是战争、饥荒、瘟疫和死亡。将它们归为一类是有原因的：或许摆脱危害最大的传染病的最有效方法，是实现世界和平和全球繁荣。遗憾的是，更广泛地了解生态学和进化与传染病的关系似乎更容易实现。

越易变化的东西，越是不变。就在我写作本书的时候，埃博拉病毒的暴发已经在西非造成数千人死亡。埃博拉病毒的出现验证了本书中提出的很多观点。埃博拉病毒是一种人畜共患疾病。病毒很可能起源于蝙蝠，虽然由蝙蝠传播给人类的情况并不常见，但对各种毒株的基因分析表明，这种情况已经多次发生。短期内无法通过技术手段解决相容筛选的问题，到目前为止，尚无针对埃博拉病毒的有效疫苗或药物治疗，但是水合作用和其他支持似乎可以改善治疗效果。隔离可以有效地关闭相遇筛选，但它本应在流行病的早期阶段最为有效。西非的后殖民地基础设施不可能，也不能单独应对埃博拉的挑战，而全世界的注意力都在其他地方。如前文所介绍的传染病一样，当全球旅行把埃博拉病毒传播到北美和欧洲时，情况就突然发生了变化。迄今为止，非洲以外地区埃博拉病毒的传播已被及时阻止。

与HIV一样，对埃博拉的恐惧让人们对这一疾病产生了阴影。感染者对家人隐瞒病情，让了解埃博拉的传播范围和动态更加复杂。人们一直在讨论，不要污名化在非洲服役后回国的国际医护人员的重要性，同时要理智地处理同胞的传染风险和对传染的恐惧。恐惧也导致了撒哈拉以南非洲疫情最严重地区的粮食匮乏，这使检疫工作更具挑战性，并造成了另外一场危机。 105

埃博拉让人们不寒而栗，一部分原因是其传播方式，另一部分原因是该病致死率极高，尤其是在非洲。埃博拉感染者的所有体液，尤其是死于该病者，都含有传染性病毒。埃博拉病毒可怕的传播方式意味着相遇筛选相对较小。人们只需要接触到一些细小的病毒颗粒就会被感染。但也正是这个原因，除了医护人员和照顾过死者的人，其他的人不太可能被感染，因为接触到被污染体液的机会很小。不幸的是，非洲的传统习俗让死者的很多亲属在葬礼前和举行期间都会接触到尸体。例如，美国第一个被确诊为埃博拉病毒感染者托马斯·邓肯死于该病，虽然他的家人在他被感染后与他共同生活了几天，却没有被感染，而在医院照顾邓肯的两名护士却被感染了。欣慰的是，经过治疗，两名护士已经康复。

撰写本书时，很难预测埃博拉疫情的蔓延轨迹。然而，读者们在阅读本书时，另一种传染病会不可避免地出现。变化很多……礼貌地向不请自来参加派对的蒙面陌生人表示歉意，并解释说，用餐之前，自己必须要洗手；向客人讲述有效接种疫苗的真实故事；遵医嘱服用药物（但请随时与医生讨论！）。我们不可能生活在一个没有传染病的世界里，但如果采取有效的防控措施，我们就能更加安全地生活。 106

索 引

（条目后的数字为原文页码，见本书边码）

L

M

N

O

P

Q

R

S

T

Marta L. Wayne and Benjamin M. Bolker

INFECTIOUS DISEASE

A Very Short Introduction

Contents

Acknowledgements

For Charlie, Norma, Tara, and (*in memoriam*) Django.

We acknowledge the partial support of the US National Institutes of Health. We would like to thank the understanding and professional editorial staff at Oxford University Press, especially Cathy Kennedy, along with our colleagues who contributed friendly reviews and technical advice: Rustom Antia, Janis Antonovics, Julia Buck, Robin Bush, Jonathan Dushoff, David Earn, David Hillis, Lindsay Keegan, Marm Kilpatrick, Aaron King, Marc Lipsitch, Glenn Morris, Juliet Pulliam, Marco Salemi, and David Smith. Needless to say, we are entirely responsible for any remaining errors or oversimplifications.

List of illustrations

Chapter 1
Introduction

We talk about 'infectious lyrics' and 'viral videos'. Metaphors of infectious disease saturate Western popular culture in the 21st century. Anxiety over the next pandemic simmers subliminally worldwide. Infectious disease crises come and go: over the past decade we have worried in turn about bioterrorism, SARS, H1N1 influenza, and the Ebola virus.

As recently as the 1970s, doctors were boldly proclaiming the beginning of the end for infectious disease. They thought their arsenal of vaccines for preventing viral diseases and broad-spectrum antibiotics for treating bacterial infections could handle any threat. But disease was never dead, or even in remission. Even as the doctors announced victory, drug resistant strains of *Staphylococcus aureus* (one of the 'flesh-eating bacteria' of British tabloids) were spreading in hospitals. (Japan had experienced outbreaks of drug resistant bacteria in the 1950s, but at the time these epidemics were little noticed in the West.) Things got worse as HIV, which has stubbornly resisted the development of vaccine to the present day, emerged in the 1980s. In recognition of the renewed threat of infectious disease, the US Institute of Medicine coined the phrase 'emerging and re-emerging diseases' in the early 1990s.

An infectious disease is one that you can catch from another person or organism as a result of the transmission of a biological agent. In contrast, you fall ill with non-infectious diseases—heart disease, diabetes, Alzheimer's—because of a combination of your environment and genes inherited from your parents. The agents that cause infectious disease are called *pathogens* or *parasites*. While biologists once used 'parasite' only to describe relatively large disease-causing agents such as tapeworms or ticks, they now include microorganisms (viruses, bacteria, and fungi) in this category as well, making the two terms more or less synonymous.

Infectious disease frightens us precisely *because* it is infectious. Its agents are usually invisible to the naked eye and thus largely unavoidable, except by entirely eschewing human contact. Edgar Allan Poe illustrated the fear of infection, as well as the futility of cutting off human contact to evade infectious disease, in his 1842 story *The Masque of the Red Death*. In Poe's story, a group of wealthy nobles withdraw to an isolated location to escape from a plague called the Red Death. Ultimately, a costumed stranger infiltrates the group at a masquerade ball. Despite their precautions, the entire group succumbs to the disease.

However ineffective it might be, for most of human history the strategy taken by Poe's nobles—avoiding disease transmission—has been the only way to combat infectious disease. Since the mechanisms of disease transmission were unknown until the mid-19th century, all human societies could do in the face of an epidemic was to cut off contact with infected areas. In 1665, Isaac Newton retreated to the countryside to avoid the Great Plague of London—and incidentally invented calculus and discovered the law of gravity. In the same year, the English village of Eyam voluntarily quarantined itself to prevent the spread of the plague, with half or more of the villagers ultimately dying. The word 'quarantine', which now describes the compulsory isolation of potentially infected people to avoid transmission to others, is derived from the forty days that ships had to wait outside the city of Venice to be sure they were free of plague.

Quarantines (at least those better than the one in Poe's story) do block transmission, but they are fundamentally reactive—they are only imposed once we become aware of a serious threat of disease. They help only healthy people living in uninfected populations, not individuals who have already been infected or uninfected people unlucky enough to be stuck in the quarantine zone. On the other hand, quarantines can be effective against any disease, provided that we know something about its mode of transmission (since plague is spread by rat fleas, preventing communication among humans while allowing rats to move freely is useless).

Quarantines are deployed to protect groups of people, rather than individuals. As medical science improved, public health officials began to shift their focus from the protection of populations to the protection of individuals. Immunization—the process of protecting people by stimulating their immune systems with foreign substances such as mild pathogen strains or toxins—was the first of several major breakthroughs in individual-focused infectious disease control. Immunization for smallpox was widely practised in Africa, China, India, and Turkey by the early 18th century. It achieved public visibility in the West following its importation to England in 1721 by Lady Mary Wortley Montagu, the wife of the British ambassador to Turkey, and more spectacularly via an 'experiment' in the same year promoted by clergyman Cotton Mather of the colonial city of Boston, Massachusetts. In the face of a smallpox outbreak, Mather and his medical colleague Zabdiel Boylston promoted immunization rather recklessly, against the will of the majority of his fellow Bostonians. Despite several deaths, the experiment demonstrated an effective alternative to physical isolation: immunization protected individuals from infection without restricting anyone's freedom of movement.

Mather and Boylston's experiment also illustrated an ethical conflict between controlling disease for the benefit of an individual and controlling disease for the benefit of an entire population. Bostonians who were successfully immunized were safe from disease, but for several days following immunization they could have transmitted the disease to unprotected individuals. Most modern immunizations involve non-infectious substances, so this particular problem is of lesser concern today, but the conflict between individual and public health is very much alive.

Most immunizations can only prevent healthy individuals from becoming infected, not cure infected people. Individual-level control of disease took another leap forward in the mid-20th century with the advent of antibiotic chemicals. First derived from common household moulds and bacteria and later synthesized in the laboratory, antibiotics could be used to cure individuals who were already infected. The possibility of curing disease also lessened the fear of quarantine, which had previously been seen as a death sentence.

Between antibiotics to cure harmful bacterial infections and a wave of new and effective vaccines to prevent diseases such as polio, measles, and pertussis, an infectious disease-free future must have seemed within reach to the public health officials of the 1970s. However, public health officials were quickly faced with proof that individual-level control fails for many diseases. Vaccines work by priming the human immune system, and thus they are much harder to develop for disease agents such as malaria or HIV that have evolved strategies for evading the immune system. Antibiotics are only effective against bacteria, not other microorganisms such as viruses or fungi (while antiviral and antifungal chemicals do exist, they are much less broadly effective than antibiotics). With the realization in the late 20th century that infectious diseases were not vanquished after all, research began to shift back towards population-level control.

So far we have divided treatments according to whether they primarily help populations (quarantine) or individuals (immunization/vaccination, antibiotics). Looking more closely, however, we can see that both antibiotics and immunization do help protect populations, as well as benefiting the individuals who receive treatment. Using drugs to cure sick people reduces the impact of infectious disease, because people who recover also stop infecting others. Thus, treating sick people can reduce transmission. Using vaccines to protect people from infection means that some potentially infectious contacts (activities by infected people such as sneezing or sexual activity, depending on the disease) are wasted on people who are protected from disease, again reducing transmission. This so-called *herd immunity* reduces the size of an epidemic even beyond the direct effects of vaccination. If we immunize enough of the population, we can reduce transmission sufficiently to stamp out an epidemic. If we can do this at a global scale, then the disease will become extinct (as in the case of smallpox, one extinction that environmentalists don't worry about).

If the problem were just that some diseases are harder to control than others, we would still be making progress, albeit slowly, in the fight against infectious disease. Modern molecular biology has provided us with a variety of new antiviral drugs, and vaccines are in development even for such difficult cases as malaria. But both humans and infectious disease agents are living organisms, and all living organisms undergo ecological and evolutionary change, making infectious disease a moving target. Our growing recognition that we (and our plagues!) are tied to the wheel of life, and our realization that individual-level approaches have failed to free us from the wheel, drives the shift in infectious disease research today.

Ecological processes

As much as we try to deny it, humans are subject to the laws of ecology. We control most aspects of our environment. Motor vehicles have replaced large predators as the leading category of violent death; we have wiped out most of our potential competitors; and we have domesticated the organisms below us on the food chain. But infectious disease still connects us to the global web of life.

The most important disease–ecology connection is *zoonosis*, the transmission of new diseases from animal *reservoir hosts* to humans: Ebola (probably from bats) may be the most spectacular example, but many of the new and emerging diseases that we haven't got a handle on come from animals: SARS, avian (H5N1) influenza, and hantavirus are a few of the better-known examples. In fact, almost all infectious diseases originate in this way, and the majority of emerging disease threats are zoonotic. Since it is difficult to vaccinate or design drugs against unknown diseases, this parade of new threats is terrifying: we don't know when a 'super-disease' might emerge.

Zoonoses are by no means new. Smallpox is thought to have moved from rodents into humans at least 16,000 years ago; measles moved from cattle to humans sometime around the 9th century; and HIV jumped from monkeys and chimpanzees to humans in the early 20th century. However, rapid human population growth and changes in land use have increased human–animal contact, whether in the tropical rainforest (HIV and Ebola) or in the temperate suburbs (Lyme disease).

As well as coming into more contact with animals, humans are moving around the planet at an accelerating pace. Contact between individuals, and thus transmission, can happen much faster and over much greater distances than when Isaac Newton escaped the plague in the 17th century or when Poe penned *The Masque of the Red Death* in the 19th century. Diseases that had previously been confined to narrow regions (generally developing countries) can rapidly expand their ranges. This is true not only for human infectious diseases, but also for diseases affecting other species whose infectious agents are transported by humans in our luggage, in the food with which we sustain ourselves during travel, or on our shoes. Human travel and commerce can spread disease indirectly, by transporting *vectors*: animals (especially insects) that transmit disease from one organism to another. For example, the international trade in used tyres is spreading *Aedes* mosquitoes, the vector of dengue fever. As well as vectors, we sometimes move the reservoir hosts of zoonoses. The first human infections of the Ebola virus outside of Africa, in 1989, came from monkeys (crab-eating macaques) that had been imported from the Philippines for animal experimentation: luckily, the particular strain involved (Ebola Reston) turned out to be harmless to humans.

Increasing movement spreads vectors and hosts to new areas; environmental change allows them to thrive in their new homes. With global climate change, animals and especially temperature-sensitive insects can invade new areas in temperate regions. Although the topic is still controversial, many climate scientists and some epidemiologists are convinced that mosquito-borne diseases like dengue and malaria are already spreading to new populations under the influence of regional climate change. An even greater impact comes from more localized environmental changes driven by human patterns of settlement and economic activity. For example, the larvae of dengue-transmitting mosquitoes thrive in water bodies as small as used tyres and household water tanks. More generally, as people in the developing world move from rural to ever-growing urban environments, they face greater sewage problems (spreading cholera and other water-borne disease) and encounter new and different kinds of disease-bearing insects.

Evolutionary processes

Ecology constantly exposes us to new epidemics, but evolution is even worse: the diseases we already know change even as we attempt to come to grips with them. As living organisms fighting for survival, infectious diseases don't accidentally escape our attempts to control them. They are actually driven by natural selection to escape. Infectious disease is a moving target that moves faster the harder we try to hit it. Disease biologists frequently invoke Lewis Carroll's Red Queen from *Through the Looking Glass*, who says: 'it takes all the running you can do, to keep in the same place'.

For every disease prevention strategy, infectious diseases have an evolutionary countermeasure. Bacteria did not evolve antibiotic resistance in response to human antibiotic use: scientists have found antibiotic resistance genes similar to modern variants in DNA extracted from 30,000-year-old frozen soil. This isn't surprising, because humans did not invent antibiotics. Rather, we borrowed or coopted them from fungi, which had evolved them as a strategy for combating bacteria. However, the widespread use of antibiotics in both medicine and agriculture has allowed bacteria that are resistant to one or more types of antibiotic to outcompete their susceptible counterparts. Other organisms, such as the protozoans that cause malaria, have also evolved resistance to the drugs used to treat them. And when HIV patients are given a single drug rather than a multi-drug 'cocktail', the virus evolves drug resistance within their bodies in just a few weeks. Pathogens evolve resistance to vaccines as well as drugs, but in a different way. Rather than resistance genes spreading within the pathogen population, *strain replacement* occurs—previously rare types that are immune to our vaccines take over the population.

Although mosquitoes have smaller populations and lower birth rates than bacteria and viruses, and hence evolve much more slowly, they too have found evolutionary countermeasures to our disease control strategies. In the developed world, DDT use was discontinued as Rachel Carson and others spread the alarm about its harmful effects on wildlife, but vector control strategies based on DDT were short-lived even in developing countries because

DDT-resistant mosquitoes evolved within a decade of the onset of mass spraying programmes.

Every aspect of infectious disease biology, not just the ability to resist or circumvent control measures, is constantly evolving. Biologists have noted that the virulence of a disease—how harmful it is to its host—is an evolutionary characteristic of the pathogenic organism. Typically mild diseases can suddenly acquire a mutation that makes them much nastier. A single mutation in the West Nile virus (WNV) that arose in the late 1990s made it far more lethal to crows, although we don't know whether the same mutation is also associated with increased virulence of WNV in humans.

Although mutations are random, evolution by natural selection is not: once pathogens mutate, their subsequent success depends on ecological conditions. Biologist Paul Ewald was among the first to point out that changes in pathogens' ecological conditions, such as a shift from direct person-to-person transmission to water-borne transmission, could favour more virulent forms of infectious diseases. The rise of global air travel may drive evolutionary as well as ecological changes in disease: some biologists have pointed out that mixing between spatially separated populations can encourage virulence.

Outlook

Given these challenges, the elimination of infectious disease—the siren song of the 20th century—seems hopelessly naïve, and approaches based solely on protecting individuals appear untenable. It would seem that we must learn to live with infectious disease, rather than eliminate it. However, we must also strive to reduce the misery caused by infectious disease. Accordingly, this century has seen a shift from attempts to eliminate the agents of infectious disease, to attempts to understand, predict, and manage infectious disease transmission at the population level. The primary tools in this new theoretical effort are not technologies of magic bullets, but instead the disciplines of ecology and evolution. Ecology, because understanding ecological relationships helps us understand cycles of transmission. Evolution, because disease agents evolve, both on their own and in response to our efforts to control them.

Chapter 2
Transmission at different scales

Transmission defines infectious disease. Transmission occurs when someone passes a disease to someone else: technically speaking, when a pathogen that was established in one host organism's body succeeds in moving into another host's body and establishing itself there.

Transmission occurs in a huge variety of ways. For example, in transmission of influenza (a respiratory disease), virus particles produced by the cells in an infected person's lungs would first be coughed or sneezed into the surrounding atmosphere. The infectious particles can survive briefly in the air or on surfaces in the environment, and thus be directly transmitted from person to person with minimal contact. The receiving person could either inhale them directly, or could pick them up by touching a surface shortly after virus-containing droplets landed there. The receiver would then transfer virus particles to their nose by touching their face; from there, the natural movement of air within their nose would move the virus into their respiratory tract. In the respiratory tract, the virus particles would enter vulnerable cells and resume their cycle of spreading from one cell to another within the host's body.

Many viruses, including influenza and diarrhoea-causing viruses such as rotavirus, can survive for days in the environment, building up on particular kinds of objects known as *fomites*. Have you noticed a sudden increase in male physicians sporting bow ties? This fashion statement is a response to health researchers' identification of standard ties as fomites. Influenza viruses can even survive for several days on banknotes, especially if they are first mixed with 'nasopharyngeal secretions' (snot), although we don't actually know whether this transmission pathway is important in real epidemics.

Pathogens whose infectious particles die almost instantaneously outside the warm, wet environment of the human body often rely on bodily fluids being directly transferred from person to person, as in the case of sexually transmitted diseases such as HIV (see Chapter 4) and gonorrhoea. While sexual contact was the most common form of fluid exchange throughout most of human evolutionary history, these pathogens can also be transmitted by more modern modes of fluid exchange such as blood transfusions or the sharing of syringes by drug users.

Other pathogens that cannot survive in the environment have evolved to use other organisms, especially blood-sucking insects and mites, as *vectors* to travel from one host to another. This strategy requires considerably more biological machinery than direct transfer between the bodies of two hosts of the same species. In the extreme case of pathogens with complex life cycles such as malaria (see Chapter 6), the pathogen goes through major transformations within the body of the mosquito vector. In fact, from the perspective of a mosquito-inhabiting malaria parasite, a human is just a convenient way to transmit itself to another mosquito.

Other infectious diseases can persist much better outside of the hosts' bodies. Diseases such as cholera (see Chapter 5), typhoid, and Legionnaires' disease can survive in water, making their way from one host to another through drinking water or air conditioning systems. Anthrax—which kills its hosts quickly, reducing the potential for direct transmission from one animal host to another—produces long-lasting spores that survive for years in the environment, infecting grazing animals years later when they ingest spores attached to soil particles. Many fungi, such as certain species of *Aspergillus*, live primarily as free-living organisms, but can sometimes grow within human hosts if they find themselves there, especially if the host has its immune system weakened by stress or infection with other diseases. (These are called *opportunistic* infectious diseases, in contrast to the *obligate* dependence of most pathogens. Opportunistic infections can live in a host if one is available, but do not require a host in order to complete their life cycles.) The amphibian fungus *Batrachochytrium dendrobatidis* (Chapter 7) is closely related to non-pathogenic soil-dwelling fungi, but is itself an obligate parasite—as far as we know it can only persist in the environment for a few weeks.

Filters for encounter and compatibility

Following the work of Claude Combes, we can break the process of transmission down into three stages: (1) transfer of infectious particles from inside the original host's body to the environment; (2) transfer of infectious particles through the environment, or through the bodies of intermediary vectors or hosts, to the receiving host; (3) transfer of particles from the environment into parts of the receiving host's body such as the blood, lungs, or liver where the pathogen can reproduce. These three stages collectively comprise the *encounter filter*.

Having made it into a new host's body, the travelling pathogen must overcome physical, biochemical, and immunological barriers in order to grow in the body of the new host. In other words, even if the pathogen can pass the encounter filter, it must also be biologically compatible with the new host; this final stage is called the *compatibility filter*. A host could close its compatibility filter by having a disease-resistant genetic mutation, such as the sickle-cell variant of the haemoglobin gene that protects against malaria. Opportunistic fungal infections are usually blocked as long as the host has a properly functioning immune system. In order to block most viral diseases, however, the host's immune system needs to have encountered the pathogen before, either naturally or through vaccination.

Both the encounter and compatibility filters must be open in order for successful transmission to occur. Public health measures can close the encounter filter and are especially important in the early stages of an epidemic. Drugs or vaccines can close the compatibility filter, but they are not always available.

Methods for closing the encounter filter include simple preventive strategies such as quarantine (see Chapter 1). They also include environmental strategies such as improved sanitation to control water-borne disease, or mosquito and tick control to stop vector-borne disease. Another class of strategies tries to convince people to modify their behaviour. These include the US Centers for Disease Control and Prevention's advice to 'Cover Your Cough' to stop influenza, as well as their suggestions for avoiding mosquito-borne diseases such as West Nile virus: stay indoors at dusk, wear long pants and long-sleeved shirts, and use insect repellent. Though changing people's behaviour is difficult, it is usually the cheapest way to control disease. You don't need to inject or swallow substances that may have harmful side effects, and behavioural changes can even protect against unknown pathogens. Avoiding exchanging bodily fluids with strangers is a good idea, even if they have been screened for all currently known diseases.

Epidemic dynamics

It's easy to understand the encounter and compatibility filters at the individual level: if you can prevent the transfer of infectious particles from the environment into your body, or if you immunize yourself to prevent the infection from taking hold in your body, you can stay safe. In order to understand the effects of these filters at the population level—for example, to decide whether an immunization programme or a quarantine will stop an epidemic—we need mathematical models. Almost as soon as biologists began to understand the mechanics of disease transmission, mathematicians started to develop models to describe the effects of the encounter and compatibility filters at the population level. As early as 1760, Daniel Bernoulli, a member of an eminent Swiss family of mathematicians and scientists, used a mathematical model to describe to what extent smallpox immunization (i.e. closing the compatibility filter for some individuals) could improve public health. Bernoulli concluded that immunization could increase the expected lifespan at birth by 10 per cent, from about twenty-seven to thirty years (the expected lifespan at birth was very short in the 18th century because of the high rate of infant and childhood mortality).

Bernoulli's model only took into account the direct benefits of immunization, thus missing the key insight of herd immunity. Immunization protects the people who are immunized, but it also reduces the prevalence of the disease and thus provides an indirect benefit to non-immunized people. To eradicate disease, you don't need to close the compatibility and encounter filters entirely (i.e. immunize 100 per cent of the people, or prevent transmission 100 per cent of the time); you just need to reduce transmission enough so that each infectious case gives rise to less than one new case. In technical terms, you need to reduce the *reproductive number*—the average number of new cases generated by a single case—to less than 1. If you succeed, then the disease will die out in the population as a whole, even if a few unlucky people still get infected.

The reproductive number depends on the biology of the disease: how quickly can it produce new infectious particles? How well do they survive in the environment? It also depends on the ecology and behaviour of the host, which controls the encounter filter: how dense is the population, how do hosts interact with each other, and how often do they interact? Finally, it depends on the fraction of the population that remains susceptible to the disease, which declines over the course of an epidemic as individuals first get infected and then recover (typically becoming immune, at least temporarily) or die. To ignore this last complication, epidemiologists focus on the *intrinsic reproductive number*, R_0 (pronounced 'R-zero' or 'R-nought'), which is the number of cases that would be generated by the first case in a new outbreak. R_0 is a basic measure of disease biology and community structure; it doesn't depend on how far the epidemic has spread through the population. If you can close the compatibility and encounter filters far enough to reduce the intrinsic reproductive number to less than 1, then you can not only control an epidemic in progress, but prevent the disease from getting started in the first place.

The importance of this kind of average-centred, population-level thinking in disease control was first appreciated by Ronald Ross, who built mathematical models of malaria transmission to prove that malaria could be eradicated without completely eliminating mosquitoes, by reducing mosquito populations below a threshold level—so that on average each infected human led to less than one new human case. (As we will see in Chapter 6, mosquito control and other methods for closing the encounter and compatibility filters have successfully eradicated malaria in some places, but not worldwide.) Ross won the Nobel Prize in 1902 for elucidating the life cycle of malaria, but his biography at the Nobel Foundation's website states that 'perhaps his greatest [contribution] was the development of mathematical models for the study of [malaria] epidemiology'.

Ross's model was one of the first *compartmental models*, which divide the population into compartments according to their disease status and track the rates at which individuals change from one disease status to another. The most common, simplest compartmental model is called the *SIR model* because it divides the population up into *Susceptible*, *Infective*, and *Recovered* people. Susceptibles are people who could get infected, but are not currently infected (i.e. their compatibility filter is open); infectives have the disease and can transmit it (i.e. they are *infectious* as well as infected); recovered people have had the disease and are at least temporarily immune.

The original compartmental models spawned many variations: for example, SIS models represent diseases such as gonorrhoea where individuals go straight back into the susceptible compartment once they have been cured of disease (say by taking antibiotics), because there is no effective immunity. Dozens of books and thousands of scientific papers have been written about compartmental models. Although the original versions were very simple, researchers have since added all kinds of complexity, accounting for the effects of genetics, age, and nutrition on the compatibility filter, and constructing various representations of social and spatial networks to model the encounter filter. Compartmental models also form the basic structure of huge computer models that track the behaviour and infection status of every individual in the US population in order to understand the spatial spread of influenza epidemics.

While realism and faithfulness to the biological facts of a given disease are important, compartmental models have remained the workhorse of epidemiological modelling because, even in their simpler forms, they capture most of the important characteristics of the spread of disease through a population. Especially when we are ignorant of important information about a disease—a situation painfully familiar to epidemiologists—an oversimplified model can be more useful than an overcomplicated one, as long as we interpret its conclusions cautiously.

Compartmental models typically assume that everyone in the population starts out equally susceptible to a particular disease (at birth, or in the case of sexually transmitted diseases, once they become sexually active). Susceptibles get infected by mixing with infected people in some way—for example, being coughed or sneezed on or exchanging bodily fluids. In general the infection rate increases with the proportion of infected people in the population, but the details vary enormously among models. After an *infectious period* during which they spread disease, infected people recover; they move into the recovered compartment and gain effective immunity to the disease. As we have seen, a huge number of variations on this model are possible, including subdividing the population by age, sex, or geographic location; allowing people to return to the susceptible class from the recovered class after some time period; or allowing for variation in the rate at which different individuals transmit disease.

Even without going into any of the underlying mathematics, the structure of the SIR model (Figure 1) helps categorize the ways we can control epidemics. The most common control strategy—closing the compatibility filter by immunization or *prophylactic* drug treatment (i.e. giving people drugs to prevent rather than cure disease)—moves individuals directly from the susceptible to the recovered compartment without passing through the infected compartment on the way. Almost all other epidemic control measures affect the encounter filter in one way or another. For epidemics in wildlife or domestic animals and plants, killing susceptible or infected individuals (*culling*) removes these individuals from the population entirely, hopefully reducing R_0 below 1. Culling is one of the few available strategies, albeit a very controversial one, for controlling the foot and mouth disease virus in cattle. Post-exposure treatment increases the rate at which individuals move into the recovered compartment, importantly shortening their infectious period and reducing the number of susceptibles they can infect. Finally, transmission controls such as quarantines block infection without moving individuals between compartments.

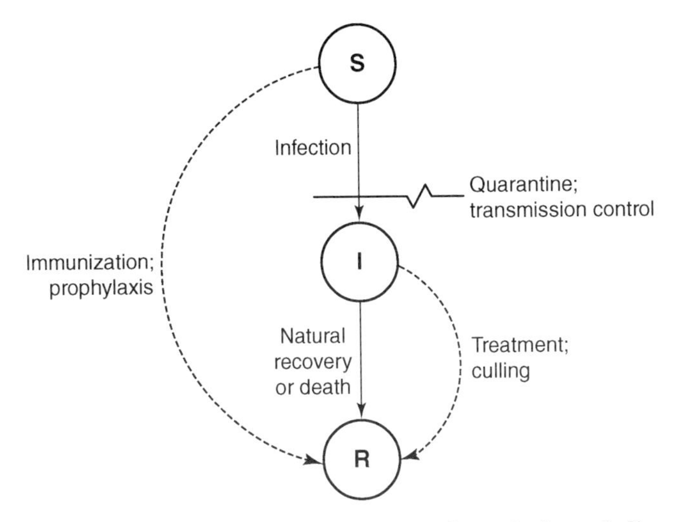

1. The SIR model describes the progression of people through disease stages from susceptible to infectious to recovered. Interventions such as culling, treatment, or quarantine can speed up or prevent transition among compartments.

As well as a conceptual framework for thinking about disease control measures, the SIR model also provides a quantitative framework for calculating exactly how much control is necessary to eradicate a disease, or how much a given level of control will reduce the level of disease in the population. Suppose we can eliminate some fraction of effective contacts, by a *control fraction* (p), by closing either the compatibility filter (e.g. by vaccination) or the encounter filter (e.g. by providing condoms or clean needles). Then the value of R_0 will be reduced by a factor $1 - p$; if R_0 is initially equal to 4 and we can achieve a control fraction of 0.75 or 75 per cent, then we will reduce R_0 to $(1 - 0.75) \times 4 = 1$.

A little bit of algebra shows that in order to reduce R_0 to less than 1 we need to increase the control above a critical value of $p_{crit} = 1 - 1/R_0$ (Figure 2). This tells us immediately why it was much easier to eliminate smallpox ($R_0 \approx 6$, $p_{crit} \approx 0.8$) than it has been to eliminate measles ($R_0 \approx 15$, $p_{crit} \approx 0.95$), despite the fact that cheap and effective vaccines are available for both diseases,

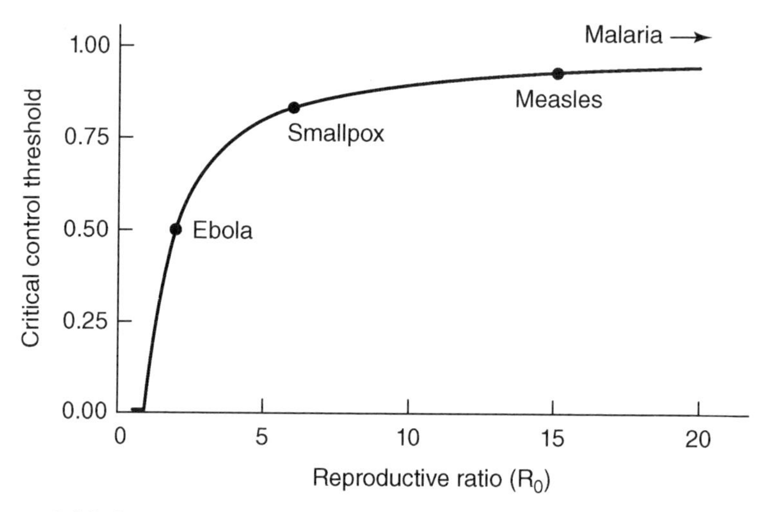

2. Critical control level required (proportion immunized or treated to prevent transmission) to eradicate an infectious disease, based on its R_0 value.

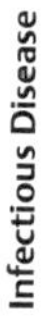

and why it will be extremely difficult to eradicate malaria, even once we have an effective vaccine: R_0 is estimated to be greater than 100 in some areas, so the critical control fraction will be greater than 99 per cent. In fact, the only way to eradicate malaria in high-disease areas will likely be to combine several different strategies (e.g. vaccine and mosquito control), each of which could have (say) 90 per cent effectiveness, so that their combined efficacy could reach the 99 per cent level that might be required.

In principle, if disease control measures can reduce R_0 below 1, they will not only terminate any existing epidemic, but will prevent recurrence of the epidemic as long as the control measures are maintained. Eradicating a disease within a given region, such as the UK or Europe, reduces the local burden of infectious disease, but does not eliminate the need for disease control unless public health authorities can somehow be 100 per cent sure that they can prevent the importation of disease from outside the eradication zone. Only if we can eradicate a disease globally, as has so far been done only for smallpox and rinderpest (a lethal cattle disease closely related to measles), can control measures safely be discontinued. This makes eradicating a disease, rather than simply controlling it, an attractive policy option—once the disease is completely gone, any resources that went into managing it can be freed for other disease control efforts, or for other societal goals.

Of course, knowing R_0 does not tell us everything about controlling disease—diseases such as influenza ($R_0 \approx 2 - 3$) and HIV ($R_0 \approx 2 - 5$) are harder to control than their relatively low R_0 values would suggest. Sometimes treatments are unavailable, or too expensive. In other cases, treatment or control measures are only partly effective. With a vaccine that is only 50 per cent effective, comparable to the experimental malaria vaccines currently being tested, and better than the best HIV vaccines available ($\approx$ 30 per cent effective), twice as many people need to be treated (if $R_0 > 2$ it would be impossible to eradicate the disease with this vaccine). Another problem is that infections may be hard to detect, and thus be out of reach of disease control efforts, for either biological or cultural reasons. Biologically, some individuals (carriers) can be infected and spread a disease while showing no symptoms; culturally, many diseases carry a stigma that makes people hide the fact that they are infected. During the ongoing West African Ebola epidemic, one of the major concerns about imposing harsh control measures is that they may simply encourage people exposed to Ebola to hide from authorities.

Compartmental models tell us much more than the level of control necessary to eradicate disease locally or globally. They also give a simple formula for the number of people who will be affected by a disease outbreak in the absence of control, or the size of the susceptible population at equilibrium for a disease that becomes established in the population. Compartmental models have also helped epidemiologists to think about the dynamics of disease—the ways that the infected population changes over time.

For example, one of the first applications of compartmental models explained that observed multi-year cycles of measles epidemics did not necessarily mean that a new genetic type was invading every few years; rather, disease spread so fast that the susceptible population was exhausted and required several years to build up to the point where it could support another major outbreak. Similarly, mathematicians have pointed out that vaccination campaigns that fail to eradicate a disease allow the number of susceptibles in the population to build up. Even if vaccination coverage stays high, these build-ups may lead to large outbreaks several years after the beginning of the campaign. Without this dynamical insight, the outbreak could easily be interpreted as a sudden change in the effectiveness of the vaccine or the transmissibility of the disease, rather than as a straightforward consequence of a sub-critical level of control.

Within-host disease dynamics

One of the many biological details that compartmental models omit in their quest for simplicity is any description of the way that disease plays out within an individual host. In compartmental models, hosts are either infected or not; we don't keep track of the level of infection within an individual (e.g. the number of virus-infected cells or the density of the virus in the bloodstream), nor of the response of the individual's immune system to the disease.

Standard compartmental models are best for understanding small pathogens (*microparasites*) such as viruses, bacteria, and fungi; because these types of pathogens tend to build up very quickly within a host, and trigger similar immune responses in most hosts, characterizing hosts as either infected or uninfected is a reasonable simplification. In populations infected with *macroparasites*—larger parasites such as tapeworms or ticks—the number of parasites per host varies greatly among individuals.

To account for this variation, mathematicians have had to design more complex models. Within the last decade or so, however, these distinctions have begun to blur as researchers build more elaborate microparasite models that track changes in the numbers of infected particles or cells and the level of activation of the immune system within an individual. For example, a large fraction of HIV transmission occurs within the first month of infection. If we want to understand and predict HIV epidemics, we obviously need to use models that distinguish between recently- and not-so-recently-infected people; we might even want to track the precise level of virus in the blood and other bodily fluids of an infected person.

Nested models, which track both changes in the number of infected people and changes in the number of infected cells within individuals, are mathematically complex—one can imagine the difficulty of keeping track of all of the virus particles within every individual in a population! Somewhat more manageable are within-host models, which focus on the progress of disease within a typical person, ignoring how the disease is spreading among individuals. Where epidemiological models represent the progress of disease in a population, and give insight into the impact and control of disease at the population level, within-host models can help understand how disease works within a single individual.

Despite this difference in scope, however, epidemiological models and within-host models have striking similarities (Figure 3). The compartmental model can easily be adapted for within-host models, especially for parasites such as viruses that must invade host cells in order to reproduce. Instead of assuming that infection builds up quickly and characteristically within individual hosts so that we can practically treat them as either uninfected or infected, we now assume that the level of infection (e.g. the number of virus particles) builds up quickly and characteristically within host *cells*. The concepts of encounter and compatibility filters are just as useful on the within-host as the within-population levels,

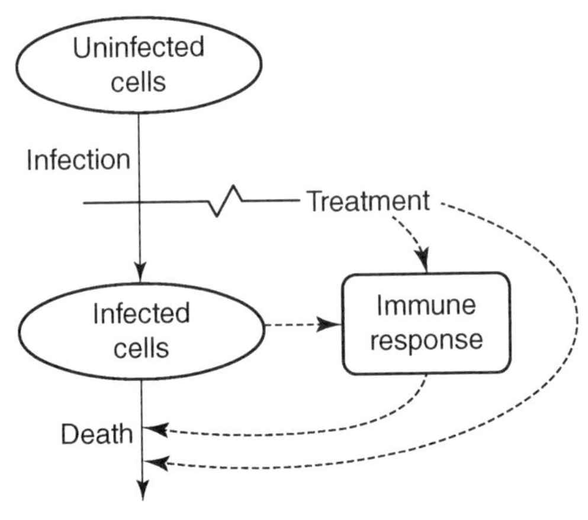

3. A within-host compartmental model showing: the infection of cells and death of infected cells; triggering of the immune response by infected cells and by treatment; killing of infected cells by the immune response and by treatment; and blocking of between-cell transmission by treatment.

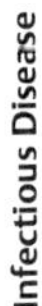

describing how infection gets from one cell to another and what prevents or allows infection of a cell by a disease particle.

Within-host models often add a new compartment to keep track of free-floating infectious particles outside of cells, and they often include a separate term for the level of immune defences activated within a host. Within-host models usually assume that the strength of immune defences increases as the number of infected cells increases. If the immune response is rapid enough and strong enough, these models show how the immune system can naturally overwhelm an infection, although not necessarily before the infection has had time to proliferate temporarily and infect another host. Within-host models can also show how drug treatments can slow down disease spread within the host sufficiently for the immune response to eradicate the disease. In viruses such as HIV and the human T-lymphotropic virus that attack immune cells, within-host models show exactly how these diseases pervert the normal immune strategy; the immune system responds to the presence of virus infection by activating more immune cells, which in turn provide more resources for virus growth. This is like finding out that you're trying to put out a fire with gasoline instead of water.

Virulence, resistance, and tolerance

Compartmental models have been used most often for widespread diseases where nearly everyone in the population is equally susceptible, such as measles, polio, or smallpox. Humans do vary in their susceptibility to infection: because they have different genotypes (i.e. complete sets of genetic material), or are better or worse nourished, or are more or less stressed. They also vary in infectiousness, how badly they suffer, and how likely they are to die from the disease. However, for the purposes of epidemiological planning it's often wise to ignore these details, at least initially.

When we turn to thinking about evolution, this variation becomes not just dangerous to ignore, but central to the questions we are asking. In the last few decades, epidemiological modellers have turned from just trying to understand how diseases spread in populations over timescales from days to years, to trying to understand how diseases evolve over timescales from years to thousands of years. What is it about the combination of a particular host, a particular parasite, and a particular environment that allows the parasite to infect a host? What determines whether the host is badly harmed by the infection or only has mild symptoms?

We have to make several important distinctions about the characteristics of parasites. The first is between infectiousness (how easily the parasite can infect the host) and virulence (how severely it affects the host if it succeeds). We often treat infectiousness and virulence as fixed properties of a parasite. Smallpox has much more horrible symptoms than measles, and a much higher chance of killing the host, regardless of the particular genetic makeup of the parasite or of the host it infects. Measles is always more infectious than smallpox, which is more infectious than HIV or Ebola. In principle, however, we can imagine two parasite strains and two kinds of hosts that 'cross over' in their effects, with one parasite having higher virulence on the first host genotype than the second and the other having higher virulence on the second genotype.

Hosts could control the infectivity and virulence of the pathogens attacking them in two ways. If the host is able to close the compatibility filter partially or completely, we say that it *resists* the parasite. As a result the parasite might not be able to infect the host at all, or it might not be able to build up its population within the host to very high levels, so that the host suffers few ill effects. Alternatively, the host might allow the parasite to infect it (or more precisely it might not invest energy in defending itself), but it could evolve mechanisms so that it was not badly harmed by infection: in this case, we would call the host tolerant rather than resistant.

Tolerance and resistance have similar outcomes at the level of the individual host (the host isn't harmed by the parasite), but very different outcomes at the level of the population. If some individuals are highly susceptible (neither resistant nor tolerant), then the presence of resistant individuals will help them by lowering the overall chances of infection, while tolerant individuals will increase the chance of infection. This is one reason that epidemiologists worry about the introduction of partially effective vaccines. If pathogens evolved to replicate more quickly within the host in order to overcome partial resistance in vaccinated people, they might increase their virulence in non-vaccinated people; if vaccination makes people tolerant rather than resistant to disease, they could still spread infection to unvaccinated people.

Chapter 3
Influenza

Unless you are lucky or very careful, you have probably had influenza (the flu) sometime in your life. Flu is familiar to almost everyone, occurring in every country, every year. It has been with us throughout history. Though not as gruesome as some viral diseases such as Ebola, the flu virus has caused more deaths than any single disease outbreak since the Black Death (bubonic plague) of the 14th century: twenty to fifty million people worldwide died from the 1918 Spanish Flu.

Furthermore, although non-epidemiologists may not think of it as a big problem, the annual flu epidemic that occurs every winter in temperate parts of the world infects millions of people. Although influenza kills only a small fraction of even the frailest elderly population, it is still thought to cause as many as 40,000 deaths in the US in a typical year (not a pandemic year). Because influenza causes many deaths indirectly, e.g. due to secondary infections, these numbers are estimated indirectly by estimating how many extra deaths are observed in years with large seasonal epidemics.

Influenza is even scarier in years, such as 2009, when we think we might be on the verge of a deadly pandemic that could cause millions rather than tens of thousands of deaths. Pandemics arise under very particular circumstances, but the two most important ingredients are lack of existing immunity (an opening in the compatibility filter) and virulence. If the virus has radically changed its appearance, more people than average will be susceptible because their immunity from previous years fails to protect them against the new strain. This drives the value of R_0 (the intrinsic reproductive rate, see Chapter 2) higher than in a typical year. Higher transmission is scariest if the virus is simultaneously more virulent, severely harming a larger fraction of its victims than usual. Authorities feared this situation in 2009 for three reasons: (1) the new strain was of the H1N1 type, different from the previous year's H3N2 type, which would lead to more susceptibility and a higher R_0; (2) the highly virulent 1918 pandemic was caused by an H1N1 strain; (3) the 2009 strain's virulence was initially overestimated due to biases in reporting from its origin in Mexico.

In the end the 2009 strain's virulence turned out to be about average for a flu strain overall, although it did affect younger people relatively severely, leading to more years of life lost. The 2009 H1N1 strain did officially lead to a pandemic—that is, it was a previously unobserved strain that caused significant numbers of cases all over the world—but happily it did not infect as many people, nor kill as many of them, as initially feared.

In order to prevent pandemics, we have to control transmission. Transmission can be controlled by reducing encounters (sneezing into your elbow instead of into your hand), by reducing compatibility (vaccinating to reduce the number of susceptible individuals), or ideally by a combination of both. In the 2009 H1N1 epidemic, encounter rates were reduced by closing schools throughout Mexico, as well as by discouraging large public gatherings and distributing masks and hand sanitizer. Development of a vaccine to close the compatibility filter for the new strain was swift; the vaccine became available in October 2009, a mere six months after the strain was characterized. Vaccines were initially limited, so were first distributed to the target groups believed to be most at risk, *and* to those most likely to transmit the disease, including school-age children. We'll come back to why children are an important target group for flu vaccination later in this chapter.

In first-world countries, the flu shot (or at least the ubiquitous publicity surrounding the vaccine) is as much a harbinger of winter as the shortening of the days. Unlike the measles or diphtheria vaccines that we in the developed world get once as children, we need new flu shots every year because the flu virus evolves rapidly; it changes its outer garments so fast that our immune system needs new clues each year to recognize the current disguise of this old and otherwise familiar foe.

To understand flu control, it helps to understand the evolutionary processes that lead to flu's unique capacity for costume changes. As discussed in Chapter 1, hosts and parasites are like Alice and the Red Queen in *Through the Looking Glass*: they have to run as fast as they can to stay in the same place. Hosts and parasites are locked in a race, with the host evolving to escape the parasite and the parasite counter-evolving to keep up with the host. For the host, winning the race means closing the compatibility filter so that the parasite can no longer exploit it. For the parasite, winning means keeping the compatibility filter open, so it can continue to exploit the host. Thus, 'the same place' means the parasite can still infect the host; running as fast as they can means both the host and parasite are rapidly evolving, with one trying to set itself free and the other stubbornly holding on.

It is important to remember that evolution does not always mean evolution via natural selection, the usual 'survival of the fittest' paradigm that you may remember from school. Any natural population contains organisms with many different genotypes; the current proportion of any given genotype within the population is called the *genotype frequency*. To evolutionary biologists, evolution means *any* change in genotype frequencies over time. Popular discussions of evolution mostly focus on the process of natural selection, the change in the frequencies of genotypes because of differences in fitness—i.e. the expected numbers of offspring and probabilities of survival of each genotype. But genotype frequencies can also change due to chance events, a process referred to as *genetic drift*.

To distinguish further between natural selection and genetic drift, let's consider an imaginary infectious disease. Suppose a mutation happens at random in the host genotype that confers complete resistance to the disease and has no bad side effects. If the disease is common, then the mutation should increase in frequency in the population due to natural selection; people who carry the mutation will have higher fitness in the presence of the disease, and the same fitness in its absence. However, there's a small probability that before the mutation has a chance to increase in frequency, the extended family in which it arose will decide to embark on a trip together—and be tragically wiped out in a bus crash. This is an example of genetic drift: evolution happening because of a chance event that has nothing to do with the infectious disease, the host's fitness, or the mutation itself. One of the reasons that predicting flu epidemics is so difficult even for expert epidemiologists is because flu evolves by genetic drift as well as by natural selection; chance events that happen before the temperate flu season can set the year's flu epidemic off down different, unpredictable tracks.

Evolution requires genetic variation. The ultimate source of genetic variation is mutation, a process at which viruses excel. Another important source of genetic variation is recombination, combining existing genotypes in different ways. The influenza virus takes advantage of both mutation and *reassortment*, a type of recombination. As we will explain, hosts' (i.e. humans') power to evolve by mutation is limited, but we make good use of recombination as a key feature of our immune system. The reason we can recognize so many parasites is not because our genes code a different protein (*antibody*) to recognize each one—our genomes would have to be many times their already huge size. Instead, we reuse the same small pieces of genes in different combinations to create a range of antibodies. These different antibodies recognize specific parts of the costumes, which are known as *antigens*, of many different parasites.

Our genomes are made of DNA that is replicated or copied by a special protein called a *polymerase*. Our DNA polymerase not only copies DNA, it also proofreads the new strand being produced, and can correct many of the errors inevitably made during the copying process. The influenza virus has a genome coded in RNA rather than DNA. It also encodes its own RNA polymerase. However, unlike the polymerase that we produce to replicate our DNA, flu's RNA polymerase cannot proofread to correct replication errors. As a result, replicating flu viruses end up with many more errors—that is, mutations—in the new copies of the genome. The virus arising from the new, mutated RNA genome will have the mutation, and so will its offspring. The result is that mutation rates for flu are 100,000 times greater than our own. Because flu mutates rapidly, it evolves rapidly.

Mutations in influenza lead to *antigenic drift*, a process of slow change in the flu virus over time. Under antigenic drift, our bodies can sometimes use the same set of antibodies to recognize strains of flu that have drifted apart. Their short-sleeved shirts may have changed from stripes to solids to plaids, but they are still recognizable as shirts. The new varieties of influenza that result from antigenic drift then evolve through both natural selection—genotypes that are slightly better than average at evading the existing repertoire of host antibodies will have higher fitness—and genetic drift. Because flu constantly evolves, both vaccinated people and unvaccinated people who contract flu naturally tend to lose their immunity after a few years.

The flu has another evolutionary trick. Its genome is divided into eight discrete segments; it can combine different variants of the segments in new ways to result in viruses with novel properties. When two different variants of the flu virus happen to invade the same cell within a host, they can reassort, trading segments of their genomes with one another to produce an *antigenic shift*. This reassortment results in fast, dramatic costume changes, effectively trading a short-sleeved shirt for a smoking jacket. These changes are hard for our immune systems to recognize, so they open the compatibility filter. As a result, the reassorted offspring have an evolutionary advantage and spread in the population—if they are also good at transmitting themselves to other hosts, overcoming the encounter filter.

Antigenic drift is not usually sufficient to cause a pandemic. The hallmark of pandemic flu is antigenic shift, particularly the reassortment of flu strains found in multiple hosts. For example, the 2009 H1N1 flu arose when different segments from viruses that were adapted to birds, humans, and swine came together in pigs.

The constantly changing costume of the flu virus consists of a protein derived from two separate genes, haemagglutinin (HA) and neuraminidase (NA). Flu strains are named for their variants of each gene: H1N1 combines HA variant #1 with NA variant #1. When a given strain of flu swaps its HA and NA genes for another type, our immune system is less able, and sometimes completely unable, to recognize the flu virus. HA and NA are antigens, the parts of a parasite that our immune system uses to recognize it. They are exposed on the surface of virus particles, where our immune system can detect them as they float in the bloodstream. When viruses infect a cell, they turn the cell into a factory for the production of more viruses; in the case of flu, the new viruses emerge from the cell by 'budding' out, rather than bursting the cell altogether. As part of the budding process, infected cells display HA and NA on their surfaces, triggering the recognition and destruction of the co-opted cells by our immune system.

There are two major types of flu vaccine. The standard flu shot (TIV) is an intramuscular injection of inactivated or 'killed' virus. A newer, less widely used type of vaccine, marketed as FluMist or FluEnz, is a nasal spray of attenuated (weakened) but 'live' virus (LAIV). (We put 'killed' and 'live' in quotes here because the consensus among biologists is that viruses are not living organisms, but the terms 'live' and 'killed' are still commonly used.) Both types contain a mixture of three different strains of virus that are predicted to be common during the upcoming flu season. Sometimes some of the same strains are included in consecutive years, if they are still common, but vaccine developers usually include at least one new strain as well, in the hopes of anticipating antigenic drift or shift.

Both TIV and LAIV trigger a response in our most common type of antibody, immunoglobulin G (IgG). IgG is sensitive to the relatively subtle changes that can occur as a result of drift. In other words, if the injection contained only versions of the virus with stripes, and mutations occur that change the costume to a solid colour, our immune system won't be able to detect the changed virus—let alone more complex changes resulting from antigenic shift, i.e. changing T-shirts to smoking jackets. It is this relatively limited ability of IgG to deal with differences in HA and NA, combined with the continuing process of antigenic drift, that requires us to get a new injection with a newly developed vaccine each year.

LAIV also triggers other parts of our immune system, immunoglobulin A (IgA) and cell-mediated immunity (CMI). IgA is another type of antibody that is present in both blood and mucus. CMI is a particularly intriguing form of immunity, not involving antibodies, which is responsible for killing any of our own cells which have been co-opted and turned into virus factories. By destroying the means of virus production rather than just cleaning up virus particles in the bloodstream (see Figure 3), CMI can potentially be far more efficient than antibody-mediated immunity.

If it is so effective, why isn't LAIV given more widely? There are two major reasons. First, and most important, TIV is more effective in generating an immune response in adults—a strong IgG response is better than a weak or absent IgA/CMI response. Second, people who receive LAIV can *shed* virus (i.e. release it into the environment where it can infect others) for a short period after vaccination. This is risky for people with weak immune systems who come in close contact with recently vaccinated people. LAIV is not recommended for people with weakened immune systems, including pregnant women, people under two or over forty-nine, and people with chronic infections such as HIV.

Modern vaccination programmes try to go beyond protecting individuals to protect the entire population. Vaccines can reduce the severity of the annual flu epidemic in several ways. First, they can prevent infection of the vaccinated person altogether. This clearly means less infection—we protect not only our vaccinated individual, but also anyone she would have transmitted disease to if she had been infected. However, even vaccines that do not completely block infection can reduce subsequent transmission. Adults who have received TIV often recover faster than unvaccinated people even when they are unlucky enough to get the flu. This is good for individuals (they suffer symptoms for a shorter time and may be able to get back to work sooner); it also cuts down on overall infection because they have less chance to transmit to others during their shortened infectious period. Vaccinated people may also shed less virus, and hence be less infectious, during the time the virus is present in their bodies. Finally, vaccinated people help control the epidemic via herd immunity (see Chapter 2): potentially infectious contacts of infected people with vaccinated people are wasted (from the pathogen's point of view), leading to a reduction in R_0. If we can successfully immunize enough people (more than a proportion $1 - 1 / R_0$), then infectious people will generate fewer than one new case each and the virus will go extinct.

It is important to prioritize whom to vaccinate first, particularly if vaccine supplies are limited, as was the case early in the 2009 H1N1 outbreak. Even when there is enough vaccine to go around, it is important for public health agencies to decide whom to target with advertising and outreach. One obvious choice is to concentrate on people who are most at risk of severe disease or death. However, many of these people are vulnerable precisely because they have weakened immune systems, which means that vaccination may not protect them even if they can be convinced to get the shot. Another, complementary approach is to focus on vaccinating the people who are most likely to transmit the virus.

Epidemiologists use contact networks to identify individuals within populations who have high transmission rates. Contact networks focus on the 'encounter' stage of transmission—if an uninfected person doesn't encounter an infected one, transmission won't happen. Figure 4 shows a middle-class family in the US, consisting of two parents, two children, and one grandparent. One parent works outside the home in a small business with three other co-workers, while the other parent has an online business and spends a lot of time working in the local coffee shop with a business partner. The two children, aged five and seven, attend the local elementary school. Each child has ten classmates plus one teacher. The grandparent lives independently but near the family's home, and comes over for dinner several times a week.

Casual interactions like saying hello to people only occasionally result in flu transmission. The most important encounters for flu involve regular physical contact, or opportunities for sneezing on and being sneezed upon. Each such contact, for each member of our core family of four, is shown as a line in the figure. This simplified (but not unrealistic) example shows that the children

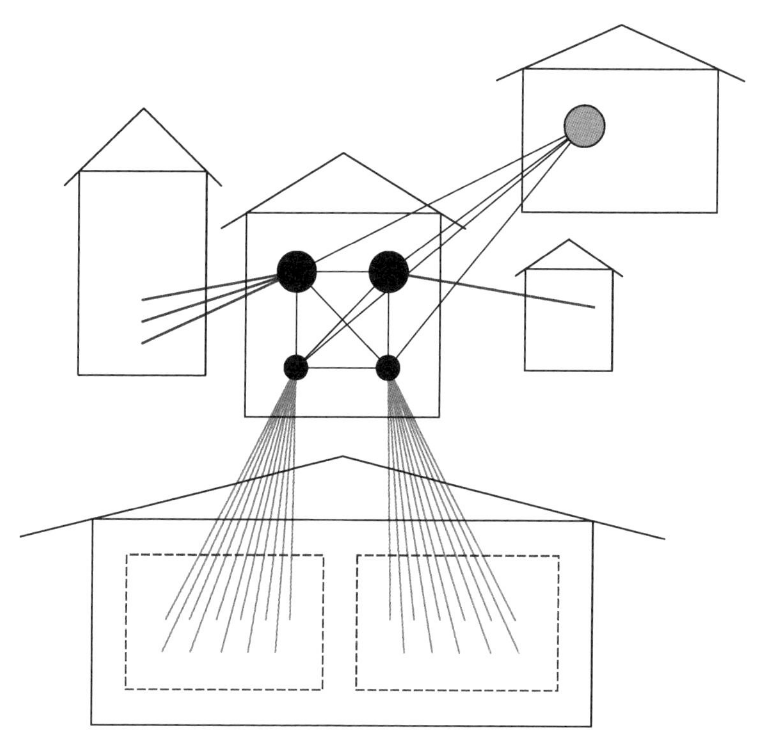

4. Contact network for a Western middle-class family consisting of two parents, two school-age children, and one grandparent living independently.

have the highest number of epidemiologically meaningful encounters. By extension, they are the most likely to bring disease into the family, particularly to the grandparent, who is the most likely to have complications from the flu. For this reason, vaccinating kids is a high priority not only to protect them, but also to protect the elderly. Obviously, contact networks vary considerably from one region to another, as well as by socio-economic status within regions, so careful comparative work is required to set global vaccination priorities.

Flu also represents an interesting case study for an age-old debate: are some kinds of research too dangerous to allow? If people do go ahead and conduct this research, should the results be available only to a limited, carefully screened subset of researchers and policymakers, or should scientific knowledge be available to all?

Scientific research is funded by governmental organizations, non-governmental organizations (NGOs), and industry. Industrial research is usually proprietary—it is kept private so that companies can get a return on their investment. But research funded by governments and NGOs is science for the people. The results of such work should be available to all, particularly when the research is ultimately paid for by taxes and charitable contributions and is directly relevant to human health.

Unfortunately, some of the same research that helps predict pandemics could also be used for nefarious purposes by bioterrorists. Such 'dual-use' research is subject to international treaties and export restrictions. Even if it is not deliberately misused, terrible things could happen if laboratory-developed super-strains accidentally escaped the confines of research labs.

The most critical indicator of pandemic flu—what determines whether a new combination of HA and NA types from avian, porcine, or human sources can spread widely in human populations—is the route of transmission. Flu becomes pandemic only if efficient human-to-human transmission is achieved—specifically, airborne transmission. Thus, an important public health priority is to understand how airborne transmission between humans could evolve and what identifiable hallmarks we should be looking for in order to be able to detect emerging pandemic strains before they spread very far.

Flu research during the first two decades of the 21st century resulted in a face-off between people who embraced the democratization of knowledge and people who feared misuse of that knowledge. The primary motivation behind the controversial research is simple: if we can understand what genetic changes make pandemic flu different from routine seasonal flu, specifically what changes are required to allow airborne transmission, we can potentially see a pandemic strain coming and take appropriate precautions. Maximum response to every case of flu is not an option, because resources are finite and because we value individual freedoms as well as public health. Thus, extraordinary control measures should only be taken when risk is high, but how can we know when that threshold has been crossed?

Flu research became extremely visible in 2011 not because of breakthroughs in understanding pandemics, but because of controversy over the publication of two high-profile papers about airborne transmission. Scientists were studying how H5N1, a particularly virulent strain of avian flu, could achieve airborne transmission from one ferret to another. Ferrets are an important model animal system for studying flu transmission in humans, in part because, like people, ferrets sneeze when they are infected with flu.

The road to publication of this research was long and rocky. The papers were originally submitted in August of 2011. Four months later, the US National Security Advisory Board for Biosecurity initially recommended that key details of the experiments be omitted from the two papers to address security concerns. In May of 2012, the first paper was finally published online, having languished for two months following acceptance. The second paper came out in late June of the same year, and was pithily referred to by *This Week in Virology*, a popular podcast, as 'the second ferret of the apocalypse'. The path to uncensored publication was cleared once experts around the world decided that the potential public health benefits of publication, with all the details, outweighed the potential harm.

One particularly interesting aspect of the controversy is that in the winter of 2012 scientists themselves agreed to a moratorium on *gain of function* research on H5N1—research that tries to create highly virulent forms of pathogens—until concerns and proper safeguards could be discussed. The 2012 moratorium had initially been proposed to last for sixty days, but ultimately lasted almost a year. Such self-imposed restrictions are rare, but are critical to maintaining public confidence in science. However, in October 2014 the US government issued a new moratorium banning funding of new research on gain of function, not because of fears of bioterrorism but because it was discovered that the key US government research centres had mishandled potentially dangerous samples of other pathogens.

The 'two most famous papers almost not published' found that HA, one of the two most important garments involved in flu's costume changes, determines both how transmissible *and* how virulent a particular strain of flu is likely to be. For example, some forms of HA such as those found in H1N1 can infect human cells via proteins found on the surface of cells in our noses and throats. These forms are highly transmissible, because the virus can easily find its way in and out of new hosts when it doesn't have to travel very far into our bodies. But H1N1 is not highly virulent, because the virus does not usually find suitable cells to infect deep in our lungs, and is thus less often associated with pneumonia. Other forms of HA, such as H5N1, encounter appropriate cells only deep in the lungs. They can therefore cause damage leading to pneumonia, and so are far more virulent. However, transmission of this dangerous strain is low because H5N1 particles can't infect us unless they find their way far down into our lungs.

Thanks to the now published research on ferrets, we know that only a small number of mutations are required for H5N1 to evolve the capability for airborne transmission between humans—at least for the particular strain of H5N1 virus that the researchers studied. Moreover, we are pretty sure what those mutations are. We have identified the costume change that this particular strain of virus would likely perform if it were to become pandemic—and thus we could recognize it *before* a major outbreak. If these signature mutations are found in all airborne strains, then we can detect when flu is on the path to becoming airborne (and hence likely pandemic) by tracking the genetic sequences of flu samples from domestic poultry and human patients.

Why the caveats about 'this particular virus strain'? Because influenza evolution, like any other kind of evolution, depends on where you start. While we understand the ways in which the particular strain of H5N1 that was studied by the researchers could become pandemic, we don't know if we can generalize those ideas even to other variants of H5N1, let alone to different strains such as H7N9, which is currently circulating in Asia.

Regardless of one's personal opinion about the wisdom or the utility of the 'two most famous papers almost not published', they have set important precedents for future dual-use research. The restraint that scientists showed while trying to decide whether to publish this research suggests that the research community, as well as world leaders, may at last be embracing the precautionary principle (scrutiny prior to any negative consequences, rather than after the fact). It also suggests that scientists realize that the active engagement of a broad array of stakeholders is essential to maintaining public trust in science.

Chapter 4
HIV

Our second case study is HIV, another virus likely to be familiar to most readers. HIV is the human immunodeficiency virus that causes acquired immunodeficiency syndrome, or AIDS. Once a person is infected with HIV, they may live for many years without showing any symptoms, but are still capable of transmitting the virus. After some time following the initial infection (usually several years), the virus population within the infected person begins to increase rapidly, ultimately causing immune system collapse. The HIV positive person then becomes vulnerable to opportunistic infections (see Chapter 2)—infections caused by disease agents such as the bacterium *Pneumocystis carinii*, which causes pneumonia, or the fungus *Candida albicans*; neither of these pathogens can infect a person with a normally functioning immune system. Certain types of cancer, such as Kaposi's sarcoma, also occur more frequently in people living with AIDS. Untreated, HIV infections are usually fatal within five to ten years. The proximate cause of death is usually opportunistic infection, rather than HIV per se.

HIV is a very different virus from influenza; it has a different mode of transmission between individuals, as well as a different evolutionary potential. HIV is transmitted in our most intimate moments, by exchange of bodily fluids. Many people think of HIV primarily as a sexually transmitted disease, because both semen and vaginal fluids carry enough virus to cause a new infection. However, our blood also carries HIV, which means that transmission can happen any time someone comes in contact with an infected person's blood. Medical personnel stick themselves with needles accidentally, and intravenous (IV) drug users share needles. Recipients of blood transfusions, especially haemophiliacs and others who need frequent transfusions, were often infected in the early days of the HIV epidemic (most blood supplies are now rigorously screened for HIV and many other blood-borne pathogens). Because breast milk also carries the virus, babies can contract HIV while nursing from their HIV-infected mothers.

Understanding routes of transmission is key to protecting both populations and individuals, who can modify their behaviour accordingly (safe sex, needle exchange programmes for IV drug users, eye protection and needle stick protocols for health workers, etc.). As we'll see later, being able to identify the most common routes of transmission also helps inform the use of limited resources for HIV treatment. But before we can understand treatment, we need to know more about HIV.

One of the biggest challenges of HIV is its extraordinary evolutionary potential. One might almost believe that HIV has a cloak of invisibility, rather than a series of costumes like influenza. The first few decades of research on HIV were nightmarish, because of HIV's uncanny ability to become invisible to our immune systems and to our treatments. We could not develop vaccines, because the virus changed too quickly—much more quickly than influenza, whose costume changes on the scale of years are problematic enough! That evolutionary prowess also means that HIV is incredibly variable around the world. So, in trying to create a vaccine, we would not be tracking just one moving target, but many. We feared we would never be able to develop a drug with lasting efficacy, because HIV seemed to effortlessly become invisible to our medicines as well. In order to understand HIV, then, we have to understand the details of how this pernicious disappearing act works.

Part of HIV's invisibility comes through an insidious strategy: it hides inside our own genomes. HIV is a retrovirus, which means that it has an RNA genome that is first copied into DNA by a complex viral protein, *reverse transcriptase* (RT). The resulting double-stranded DNA can then be integrated into our genomes by means of another viral protein, *integrase*. The fact that HIV can become 'us' is one of the reasons it is so difficult to cure.

However, HIV can only enter certain types of cells, an example of the compatibility filter described in Chapter 2. In order for HIV to enter a cell, the cell must have surface proteins (receptors) that fit a particular knob sticking out of HIV's envelope, *gp120* (glycoprotein—a protein with sugars attached to it—with a molecular weight of 120). Thus, blocking the gp120 compatibility filter should confer resistance to HIV. Remarkably, there is a mutation in humans that does almost exactly that. HIV actually needs to use two receptors to enter the cell: the primary receptor for gp120, which is called CD4, and a co-receptor, called CCR5. Humans with the CCR5-Δ32 mutation lack the co-receptor for gp120 and are hence resistant to HIV infection. However, to have complete protection from HIV, a person must have two copies of this mutation, one on each strand of DNA. People with a single copy of CCR5-Δ32 (heterozygotes) can still be infected and become symptomatic, though they are still more resistant than people with no copies at all.

Only three cell types have the appropriate receptors to bind with gp120, and all three are part of our immune system. It is because HIV targets immune cells that infection by HIV results in immunodeficiency. The virus hides in these cells until it is activated. Once activated, the virus begins to replicate, ultimately resulting in the death of these immune cells and weakening our ability to respond to other infections.

As noted in Chapter 3 on influenza, mutations happen at random, without respect to whether or not they are going to be advantageous to the virus. The mutation rate of a virus, then, is critical to understanding how easily (and hence how frequently) any given mutation can occur. Intuitively, we might expect HIV to have a much higher mutation rate than influenza since it evolves so quickly. And HIV's mutation rate is indeed more than ten times higher than influenza's.

Interestingly, estimates of the mutation rate for HIV depend strongly on context—for example, when we measure mutation in viruses within humans, rather than in a test tube.

HIV replication uses two distinct enzymes. One is the virus's own RT, which as described previously converts viral RNA into DNA. The DNA versions of the viral genome which have been integrated into our own DNA are copied by a second enzyme, our own RNA polymerase. These new RNA genomes are then repackaged into the virus particles that emerge from one cell to infect another. Most HIV mutations come from the reverse transcription step. The HIV RT enzyme makes more mistakes than the enzyme used by influenza, so HIV's mutation rate is higher than that of flu.

Mutation is not the only source of variation for HIV. Unlike influenza, which has a segmented genome and so can combine different viral segments from multiple viruses, HIV exchanges portions of its single-piece genome with portions of the genomes of other HIV viruses, a process called recombination. However, recombination as practised by HIV is fundamentally different from recombination in organisms such as humans, fruit flies, or pea plants. Recombination happens during the reverse transcription step, when the information in the RNA is copied into DNA. The viral RT sometimes switches from one template, the viral genome being copied, to the other (and back again). This process is called template switching. To understand template switching, imagine that you were using tracing paper to trace two parallel lines, but you are only allowed to trace one line at a time. You start at the left end of one line and move to the right. Now imagine that your tracing paper shifts up or down at random, such that sometimes you are tracing the top line and sometimes you are tracing the bottom line, but always drawing from left to right. In the end, you will have drawn a single straight line, but it will contain copies of parts of both lines. Similarly, recombinant HIV genomes contain all the parts of a single genome, but recombined from two different copies.

Because of mutation and recombination, HIV is constantly changing, to the point that it seems able to become invisible. Because vaccines rely on an immune 'photographic memory' of what a pathogen target looks like, designing a vaccine against HIV has proved extraordinarily difficult, as mentioned earlier. But HIV's invisibility is perhaps most notorious in its astonishing ability to render drugs useless, because it evolves resistance so quickly within an individual host.

We have already discussed the human mutation CCR5-Δ32, which confers resistance to HIV by blocking the compatibility filter. As it turns out, the mutation was already present in human populations before the HIV epidemic. While HIV has likely been infecting humans only for about a century, the CCR5-Δ32 mutation has been found in DNA from ancient human remains. We thus have direct evidence that the CCR5-Δ32 mutation has been around for nearly 3,000 years. Because HIV is much younger than that, and because the CCR5-Δ32 mutation is common in some human populations, researchers speculated that CCR5-Δ32 had risen to relatively high frequency because it protected against some older pathogen, such as bubonic plague or smallpox. However, careful analyses of the CCR5-Δ32 gene and its surrounding DNA revealed that the high frequencies today are most likely a happy accident—the result of genetic drift rather than natural selection. Other, less well-known genes conferring resistance to HIV also appear to be far more ancient than HIV.

In contrast to resistance mutations in the human genome, the resistance of HIV to drug therapies frequently arises from new virus mutations within individual humans, though resistant strains are sometimes transmitted from person to person. Despite these challenges, a regimen of *highly active anti-retroviral therapies* (HAART), developed in the mid-1990s, is extraordinarily effective against HIV. HAART uses a combination of three drugs to reduce HIV proliferation. Generally, the drugs work to directly block HIV reverse transcription, in two different ways. One class of drugs acts by tricking the RT enzyme into incorporating chemicals that stop the extension of the RNA genome. These chemicals look like the building blocks used by RT, but function differently. Once one of these chemicals is incorporated, the enzyme can't continue synthesizing the genome. This class of drugs is called *nucleoside reverse transcriptase inhibitors* (NRTIs); two different NRTIs are usually used in HAART. The other class of drugs directly binds to the RT, stopping it from working. These drugs are called *non-nucleoside reverse transcriptase inhibitors* (NNRTI); usually only one NNRTI is used in HAART to complement the NRTIs.

The mutations that make HIV resistant to NNRTI (for example) are extremely improbable. However, even an event that is unlikely on a case-by-case basis can become common if it has sufficient opportunities to happen. Individual HIV genomes don't last long inside a human: a given HIV virion in the bloodstream survives for about six hours. Because the total number of virions is approximately constant, that must mean that virions are replaced by new ones about four times per day. In addition, each person infected with HIV has tens of millions of virions in their body. Thus there are hundreds of millions of cycles of replication, and hence opportunities for mutation, every few days. We can use a lottery analogy: if you bought hundreds of millions of lottery tickets, you would presumably eventually win the jackpot. In other words, because there are so many viruses turning over so quickly within an infected individual, even improbable mutations will happen eventually.

To understand why HAART is successful, one just needs to remember two things: first, that mutations happen at random; and second, the basic rule of probability about the co-occurrence of independent events. In order for the virus to evade HAART, it needs three independent mutations, one for each of the three drugs. Because the mutations are independent, the chance of their happening in the same individual is the product of the probability of each of them happening independently. That is, if the chance of each event were 0.5, then the chance of two such events would be 0.5×0.5, and for three, $0.5 \times 0.5 \times 0.5$. Now imagine that the probability of each individual mutation happening is much, much smaller than 0.5. Instead of 'extremely improbable', we are dealing with 'extremely improbable cubed', so that even with tens of millions of viruses and hundreds of millions of replication cycles, resistance is going to take a very long time to arise, if it ever does.

Anti-retroviral therapy was once reserved for patients with full-blown AIDS, in part because of the problems of drug resistance and limited resources. However, in 2013 an exciting new paradigm was announced by the World Health Organization: 'treatment as prevention'. Under this strategy, infected but otherwise healthy patients are given treatment to help reduce transmission. People on drug therapy have fewer circulating viruses in their bodily fluids than people who are not being treated, so people who are being treated are less likely to transmit the virus. At the level of the individual, people on treatment will remain healthier, happier, and productive for much longer. Some may never even become symptomatic.

However, HAART is a treatment, not a cure. Patients need to take the drugs every day, or the virus will start to increase again, because as mentioned earlier, there are copies of the virus hiding inside our own cells that are not affected by HAART. Indeed, interrupting therapy quickly results in virus numbers rebounding to pre-treatment levels. In order to completely cure an HIV infection, then, we would have to eradicate all the cells in our own bodies whose genomes unwittingly harbour HIV. Because the three cell types containing integrated copies of the virus are derived from bone marrow, doctors have actually tried to strategically destroy, then replace bone marrow, as is done for certain types of cancer such as leukaemia.

First, chemotherapy is used to eliminate all cells that might be infected with HIV, even though some are probably uninfected. However, this destroys key components of our immune systems, so we cannot survive for long without these cell types. So next, bone marrow from uninfected donors is transplanted into the patient, giving rise to new, uninfected immune cells. Simultaneously, aggressive antiviral therapy to destroy any viruses currently circulating in the blood is used throughout the chemotherapy and transplant process, with the goal of preventing infection of the newly produced immune cells.

In one patient, Timothy Ray Brown, the virus remains undetectable after more than four years. However, in two other patients detectable levels of HIV were present within a year following treatment. The circumstances were not identical between patients: Brown received a transplant from a donor who had two copies of CCR5-Δ32, the mutation that confers resistance to HIV by blocking the gp120 compatibility filter. The other patients received transplants from donors with only a single copy. Their new bone marrow then had only partial resistance to HIV infection.

Unfortunately, because matches between bone marrow donors and recipients are hard to get to begin with, finding a donor who is a match *and* has two copies of CCR5-Δ32 is very unlikely. For that reason alone, this treatment will never be available as a widespread cure. Moreover, the procedure requires extensive hospitalization and is thus not suitable for most of the millions of people infected with HIV. However, the significance of Timothy Ray Brown's cure is enormous, and his success will undoubtedly inspire treatments that can be used more widely. For example, the cure underscores the importance of the CCR5-Δ32 mutation, which potentially can drive new treatments based on the altered function of this gene.

One pressing question in HIV research, and in infectious disease research in general, is 'why now'? Where did HIV come from, and how did it so quickly become a worldwide threat to health and economic stability? If we can understand the answers to these questions, we may be better able to prevent or at least slow down the next emerging disease.

Researchers have used two primary tools to understand the emergence of HIV: contact networks (discussed in Chapter 3) and phylogenetic trees. A phylogenetic tree is one of the fundamental tools of evolutionary biology. It is a way of grouping organisms by similarity, which in turn (if you do it carefully) also groups them by relatedness. Figure 5 shows the phylogenetic trees for HIV and for influenza. Nowadays, most phylogenies are built using genetic information. The more recently two organisms share a common ancestor, the more closely related they are, and the more similar their genomes will be. We use phylogenetic trees to show relatedness by placing more closely related genomes closer together on a phylogeny, and placing more distantly related ones farther apart. Our ability to build phylogenetic trees relies, once again, on the random nature (and relatively constant rate) of mutation: genome similarity is assessed in terms of numbers of mutations that differ between two organisms. But we can do more with phylogenetic trees than just understand relatedness. We build phylogenetic trees because by analysing the shape of the tree, we can understand what kind of evolutionary processes have occurred, and over what time scales.

If mutations happen at similar rates in closely related species, which is almost always true, then we can estimate time simply by counting the number of mutations. If two viruses differ by seven

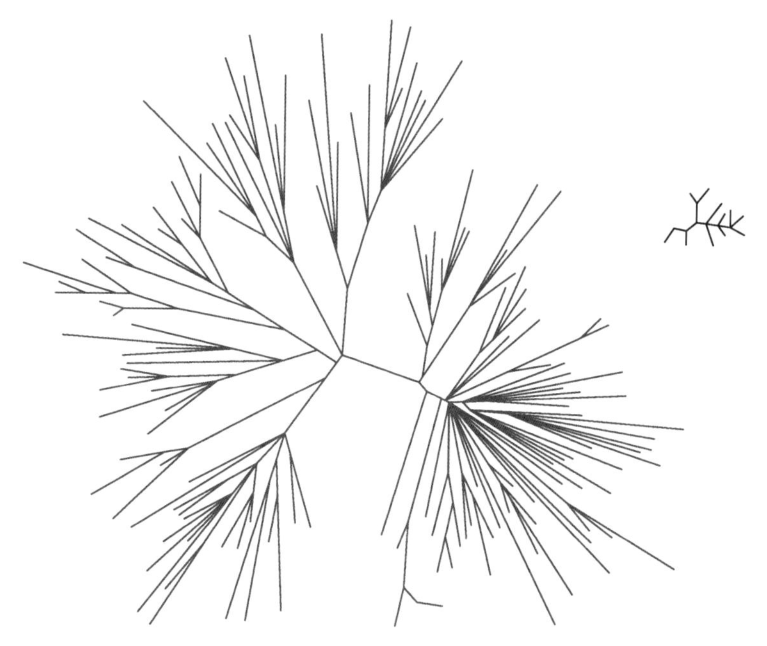

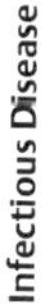

5. HIV (left, larger) is characterized by extensive genetic variation at any given time, with strains persisting for long periods of time. Influenza (right, smaller) is characterized by little variation at any given time, and strains replacing one another, rather than coexisting, over time.

mutations they are more closely related, and share a common ancestor more recently, than two viruses of the same type that vary by, say, twenty mutations. On a phylogenetic tree, the length of the branches is proportional to the number of mutations, and hence is proportional to time.

However, there's more useful information in a phylogenetic tree than just branch length: tree shape can also tell us a lot about virus evolution. Comparing a tree of influenza with a tree of HIV can give an instant intuitive understanding. The tree of influenza has a few, short branches close to the trunk. This shape reflects the fact that the majority of flu viruses do not persist in the population for long, at least not at very high frequencies. With flu, new mutants quickly take over the population, replacing old varieties. HIV trees are much more complex. It's difficult to identify a core trunk because there are so many long branches. In contrast to influenza, new mutations of HIV tend to coexist with old strains for a long time, evolving at the same time but independently.

Our best guess is that the ancestor of HIV as we know it today was contracted by some unlucky human from an infected chimpanzee butchered for food. But why did HIV become pandemic *now*? SIV, the group of viruses ancestral to HIV, has been around for thousands of years, so it seems likely that people have been exposed to them for a long time. Phylogenetic methods using both contemporary viruses and old blood samples that have been carefully stored in hospital freezers tell us that the origin of the most widespread form, the M group of HIV-1, occurred sometime between 1910 and 1930, though the original zoonotic event (the jump from chimpanzees into humans) may have occurred earlier. Other introductions of less common forms of HIV-1 occurred independently, in some cases much earlier than the M group, but these also seem to have increased in prevalence at the same time. Was something going on at that time that caused the current pandemic?

To think about this problem, we first have to understand the transfer of a pathogen from a non-human host to a human (zoonosis, see Chapter 1). Zoonoses follow two typical patterns. A zoonosis with $R_0 < 1$ in the human population, such that each human infection gives rise to less than one additional infected human, is called a spillover event. Individual infected people may be severely ill or die, but a true between-species jump or host shift won't happen because the transmission between humans is too low. On the other hand, if R_0 is even slightly greater than 1, the minimum value for persistence, then the pathogen can successfully shift hosts. Once the pathogen has started to circulate among humans, mutations may arise that help the pathogen adapt to its new host. In other words, these mutations open the compatibility filter farther and farther.

As discussed before, mutations are random; the probability of a given mutation is proportional to the number of genomes available to mutate. It is therefore critical to respond quickly to initial zoonotic events in order to limit the total mutation rate by keeping the number of human infections small. For example, in 2003 an outbreak of monkeypox virus—the first in the western hemisphere—occurred in the US as a result of a two-step host shift from a single shipment of infected Gambian pouched rats from Africa, to prairie dogs reared in captivity for the pet trade, to humans. In Africa, human-to-human transmission has evolved at least once (likely several times). However, because the patients were quickly given medical care, and because of good hygiene in the treatment facilities, human-to-human transmission did not evolve in the US and the epidemic was stopped after just seventy-one cases, with no fatalities.

The simplest argument for the current HIV pandemic, of course, is that nothing has changed—we have just been unlucky. According to this argument, the probability of SIV entering a human (passing the encounter filter) and evolving the capacity for transmission between humans (opening the compatibility filter) has been constant over time; the early 20th century just happens to be the one time it was successful. This argument is unsatisfying. Even if the probability of a successful host shift happening at any particular time is low, SIV, its primate hosts, and humans have coexisted for so long that it seems unlikely that such chimpanzee-to-human transmission has never happened before.

The most widely accepted hypothesis for HIV emergence is that successful shifts from primates to humans have indeed happened many times, but went unnoticed by the rest of the world because they failed to spread beyond the original infected community. (A similar process has happened with the Ebola virus: small outbreaks have probably been going on in isolated human populations for centuries or millennia, and have been recorded over the past forty years. It has only caught the serious attention of the West with its emergence in the urban populations of West Africa in 2014.) However, the most recent HIV shift to humans coincided with a change in human demography and sociology that facilitated transmission. This particular host shift coincided with the urbanization of Africa, which had been going on for some time, as well as the construction of roads linking many communities that had previously been isolated. Political unrest, the sexual revolution, and increased global mobility also coincided with this particular host shift.

Other researchers have argued that a simple event such as the entry of contaminated chimpanzee blood into a wound is insufficient to trigger a zoonotic shift, and that SIV got an unintentional helping hand from humans along the evolutionary road to becoming human-adapted HIV. By reusing non-sterilized syringes, medical practice may have facilitated viral persistence in humans until the mutations allowing human-to-human transmission arose.

These two hypotheses—urbanization and unsterile injections—are not mutually exclusive and may well have worked in concert to spread the virus. We will never know for certain, but by asking where HIV came from we have learned important lessons that we are already using to restrict the spread of other pathogens.

Chapter 5
Cholera

Cholera has a foundational role in any discussion of infectious disease. Cholera gave rise to Koch's postulates, one of the pillars of epidemiology. These postulates state that identifying a particular organism as the causative agent of a disease requires that (1) the organism is found in diseased people but not healthy ones, (2) the organism can be isolated from diseased people and grown in culture, (3) the laboratory-cultured organism will cause disease in a new host, and (4) the organism can be re-isolated from the newly infected host. Cholera also led to the recognition that preventive measures should focus on providing clean water, which in the process closed the encounter filter for a vast number of other water-borne pathogens.

The bacterium *Vibrio cholerae* is the cause of the diarrhoeal disease known as cholera. *V. cholerae* is a large and diverse species. New samples are assigned to types based on whether or not a particular sample reacts with antibodies produced by a mammal in response to infection by a known type. The antibodies are very specific, and only react with the type of cholera that was injected into the mammal that produced the antibodies. Thus, these antibodies can be used to identify different strains of *V. cholerae*. So, if a new sample reacts with antibodies from an animal injected with a known strain of O1, it is also an O1 type. These groups are called *serotypes*, meaning 'types based on serum', because antibodies are isolated from the blood (or serum). Two serotypes, O1 and O139, are responsible for most epidemics. Even within these serotypes, cholera bacteria can only cause epidemics if they carry at least two special genes: one to overcome the compatibility filter, and one to open the encounter filter.

To become infected with cholera, you have to ingest a huge number of the bacteria—approximately one million of them. Stomach acid, in addition to digesting our food, protects us by killing all manner of living things that we accidentally eat or drink, including cholera. Food acts to neutralize stomach acid; on a completely empty stomach, one hundred *trillion* bacteria are required to reliably produce infection in humans, 100,000 times more bacteria than when ingested with food. With that many bacteria, some can survive the gauntlet of stomach acid to make it through to the small intestine.

Bacteria that survive the stomach acid must also be able to infect cells in the small intestine. At a minimum, cholera must possess a cluster of genes involved in creating the toxin co-regulated pilus, or TCP. TCP is an essential component of the compatibility factor—without it, no illness occurs. Many other genes enhance colonization abilities, but TCP is the only one that is absolutely essential. Remarkably, even after colonization illness usually does not result unless the gene for cholera enterotoxin (CT) is expressed; that is, cholera is infectious but not virulent. Virulence and transmission are strongly correlated in cholera; CT is essential for between-host transmission of cholera (its exit strategy). CT disrupts water regulation in the intestine, producing a flood of diarrhoea that leads to dehydration and death for the host but also pushes cholera back out into the environment, allowing it to encounter new hosts.

The bright spot in all of these horrific symptoms is that treatment for cholera is remarkably straightforward. Just giving cholera victims a simple oral rehydration solution containing sugar and salt can drastically reduce death rates, or even prevent death altogether. Antibiotics are useful, but as a secondary defence. The most important benefit of antibiotics is that they shorten the infectious period, and thus can reduce the risk of transmission.

Cholera has played an important role in the history of epidemiology. Snow's discovery that cholera was spread by a contagious agent, and localizing that agent to a particular water pump during a cholera outbreak in mid-19th-century London, is arguably the first case of epidemiology as systematic detective work.

Snow's insights continue to be useful today: closing the encounter filter by setting up water purification and water treatment plants is an excellent way to prevent cholera epidemics. However, water purification by boiling (a low-tech solution that can be implemented in remote or less developed areas) requires enormous amounts of firewood, which can be dangerous to retrieve in politically unstable areas, and can lead to deforestation. Higher-tech solutions such as treatment plants or water purification via chemicals are expensive and can be logistically difficult. A recent innovation in low-tech, effective intervention is to filter water through four thicknesses of sari cloth, which can reduce infection rates by 50 per cent.

However, even with water treatment systems in place, infected people can spread cholera within their own households. Analysing the social network of cholera epidemics shows that infections spread much more rapidly within households than between them, likely due to contamination of water or food by cholera carried on the hands of caretakers. Accordingly, public health agencies have promoted water storage vessels with narrow mouths and spigots (rather than traditional open-mouthed buckets) so that infected people cannot contaminate the household's supply by dipping their hands or clothes in the water. Such interventions have reduced cholera transmission rates by almost 40 per cent.

How does cholera evolve? In the Red Queen race against hosts, bacteria generally use complete costume changes less often than viruses do. Because the biochemical machinery of bacteria differs significantly from ours, we can fight back by trying to poison the bacteria with antibacterial compounds borrowed from other organisms such as fungi (Chapter 1). This strategy usually fails on viruses, because they use so many of our own biochemical pathways that we would be poisoning ourselves at the same time. Another reason for the difference is that because bacteria mutate many times slower than viruses, they can't accumulate individual changes fast enough to hide effectively from our immune systems. Instead of evasion, they focus on resistance to host countermeasures.

Rather than switching their entire wardrobe, bacteria such as *V. cholerae* accessorize by gaining (and losing) accessories (countermeasures) according to the demands natural selection makes of them at any given time. If natural selection demands a feather boa, and one is available in the costume box (i.e. the local environment), any bacterium that picks it up will prosper. That is, the bacterium with the boa will have more descendants than the ones without it—natural selection in the usual sense. However, to a bacterium even a feather boa is heavy, so if it is not explicitly required for survival it is in the bacterium's best interest to drop it.

Obviously bacteria don't wear boas. Instead, they gain and lose genes. One way to do this is by acquiring mobile genetic elements from other bacteria. Another source of useful novel genes is from viruses that infect the bacteria. Both these mechanisms are referred to as lateral gene transfer (LGT for short), because they involve the movement of genes among organisms within generations (laterally), rather than between generations (vertically). Bacteria reproduce by dividing rather than having offspring as animals do, but the creation of new individuals isn't required for LGT, just contact between existing organisms.

One of our favourite examples of evolution in real time is antibiotic resistance in bacteria, which is usually accomplished by LGT, often via genes carried on plasmids (small circular pieces of DNA that are separate from the chromosome). Cholera is no exception. While antibiotics are not required to cure cholera, they do shorten the duration of the infectious period, and the symptoms. Heavy use of antibiotics creates a scenario where resistance will be selected, if it is present.

Unlike in viruses, drug resistance in bacteria does not generally arise as a result of new mutations, for several reasons. First, as already mentioned, bacterial mutation rates are usually much lower than viral rates—this reduces bacteria's ability to evolve new drug resistance mechanisms. Second, bacteria are more likely to trade genes among themselves—that is, participate in LGT—than viruses are. Two of the most infamous cases of drug resistance in bacteria, methicillin-resistant *Staphylococcus aureus* (MRSA) and a new scourge, carbapenem-resistant enterobacteriaceae (CRE), are caused by genes for resistance to different antibiotics.

Cholera acquires resistance primarily by gaining a piece of DNA called SXT, which is similar to a plasmid but is linear rather than circular. Once it gains antibiotic resistance, a bacterium will be more successful than one without it as long as antibiotics are in use. When antibiotic use ceases, however, resistance can be lost. Bacteria with big genomes take longer to replicate than bacteria with small ones, so bacteria containing lots of integrated antibiotic resistance genes will take longer in the absence of antibiotic to replicate than bacteria without such genes. This can be a significant handicap in a rapidly growing population, and is referred to as the *cost of resistance*.

Just as DNA can be integrated into the genome, it can also pop out again. If that happens, the bacterium with the smaller genome may have an advantage. Alternatively, if the antibiotic resistance genes are on plasmids, rather than in the chromosome itself, the plasmids themselves may be lost at random through genetic drift if they do not give the bacteria any advantage. In other bacterial systems, the cost of resistance may be driven by the metabolic costs of the resistance gene, which may make the organism expend a lot of energy pumping toxins out of its cells, or because the organism switches to a biochemical pathway that is immune to the effects of the antibiotic but less efficient at its metabolic role.

Even as cholera bacteria parasitize us, they too can be parasitized—by viruses. Remarkably, as previously mentioned, bacteria can acquire useful genes from their viral parasites—although perhaps this isn't all that remarkable when we think about it. Natural selection rewards organisms for being opportunistic, so in some circumstances a virus that gives something useful to its host is more likely to persist than one that doesn't. To understand what kind of circumstance will allow cholera to pick up genetic novelties from its viruses, we have to know a little bit more about the viruses that infect bacteria: the *phages*.

One common type of phage is the temperate phage, which can follow two strategies. The first is lysogeny: once a phage enters the cell, its DNA is incorporated into the genome of the bacterium. The phage's DNA is now called a *prophage*. The prophage is replicated along with the bacterium's own DNA, spreading to all the offspring of the original infected organism. It's a peaceable kingdom—unless the phage gets a biochemical signal that tells it that it is threatened. In that case, the phage may exit non-destructively, or it may adopt a lytic strategy.

In the lytic strategy, the phage turns its bacterial host into a virus production factory, ultimately killing the bacterium by bursting ('lysing') the cell once enough offspring are created. These new phage can go on to infect other bacteria, and pursue either the lysogenic or lytic strategy depending on environmental conditions.

As mentioned earlier, only a few strains of *V. cholerae* carry the toxin gene CT. CT is a gift carried by the temperate phage CTXϕ to its host. Once CTXϕ is ensconced in the cholera genome, the toxin can be expressed and increase transmission (and hence R_0). But phages, even temperate phages, are not altruistic. CT increases the fitness of the bacteria, but it also increases the fitness of the (now) prophage, which multiplies right along with the bacteria inside the patient's gut.

The other essential genetic ingredient for pandemic cholera is TCP, which as discussed earlier enables cholera to colonize the small intestine. TCP has another function as well: it is the receptor for the phage CTXϕ. Receptors are part of the host compatibility filter for viruses. Without the correct match between virus and receptor, infection can't occur. By expressing TCP, cholera invites infection by CTXϕ, and thereby receives the gift of CT. It's a beautiful, if sinister, example of coevolution: the two components that are necessary for high transmission of cholera (and therefore also of the prophage) are part of an interdependent system assuring the fitness of both parties.

But this pretty scenario of invitations and gifts is a profound misreading of what is more accurately viewed as an ongoing feud. The bacteria do not want the phages to come to the party, gift or no; even if the phage doesn't kill when it exits, it is still exerting a cost, however small, on the bacterium. Instead, the phage is a party crasher. It uses TCP as a receptor because TCP is something the bacterium needs for its own sake. And CT is not a gift. The phage carry it only because it increases its own fitness. If its fitness can increase along with the bacterium's, fine, but the only reason it works that way is because the phage is integrated into the bacterial genome, and so their fitness is inextricably linked. But if a mutation or new chunk of DNA were to appear that increased viral fitness still further at the expense of the bacterium, or that allowed the bacterium to maintain CT while getting rid of the rest of the party-crashing prophage, natural selection would optimize such changes and all illusions of polite society would vanish.

In fact, there is evidence for the darker version of this story. Digging a little deeper, researchers have learned that the genes coding for CT are probably a recent acquisition by the phage. There are numerous related phages that do not carry CT, but still use TCP as their receptor. Moreover, the composition of the CT genes suggests that the CT genes are newer than the rest of the genome. Not only bacteria, but also the viruses that parasitize them, can accessorize for their own benefit.

Why hasn't TCP evolved so that the CTX phage can't use it, particularly since many of these phages don't even bring CT with them? Phage infection probably doesn't hurt the cholera bacteria very much—even when threatened, this phage exits the cell without killing it. So there's little selective pressure for the bacteria to resist infection by altering TCP, especially given that they need TCP for intestinal colonization.

Other phages that infect cholera behave more like traditional predators which always kill their prey. These phages are *obligately* lytic; they can only survive by lysing or bursting their host. In other words, if they infect a bacterium, it's doomed. The best known of these lytic phages are known as the JSF phage group; they use a different receptor from CTXϕ to gain entry to the cholera bacteria.

In regions where cholera is endemic, epidemics occur seasonally. Scientists have recently noticed that epidemics in the Ganges River Delta tend to start when there are lower numbers of lytic phages in the water and stop when there are more lytic phages. Moreover, the relative abundance of phage in patients with cholera reflects their relative abundance in the aquatic environment: fewer lytic phages in patients early in the epidemic, more later in the epidemic. These observations suggest that lytic phage epidemics among cholera might ride along on top of the cholera epidemic occurring in humans, possibly even helping to control the epidemic.

Phages could be used to control cholera in individuals as well as at the population level. This form of treatment—phage therapy—has been around at least since the 1920s, when it was developed as a treatment for dysentery, a diarrhoeal disease like cholera that is caused by a different bacterium. The big advantage of phage therapy is that many phages are specific to a particular bacterium: there are no side effects. Conventional antibiotics attack not only unfriendly bacteria but also the essential bacteria in our bodies; many women have had the experience of suffering from yeast infections when antibiotics have knocked out the bacteria that normally inhabit their reproductive tracts. Successful, well-designed phage therapy would kill the bad bacteria while leaving the good guys alone.

The downside of phage therapy is that it tries to harness a living system that is capable of evolution. Once phages are introduced to a patient, they can evolve in any way natural selection directs them, including in ways that could make people sicker, as in the case of CT. One possible safeguard that could reduce such risks of phage therapy is to limit therapeutic phages' capability to exchange genes with the bacteria they infect. Phage evolvability may be one reason that phage therapy has not been embraced outside of Russia and Georgia, though very few adverse incidents involving phage therapy have been reported in the last sixty years. Phage therapy is enjoying a resurgence of interest around the world, in part due to the rise in antibiotic resistance, but also in part due to the apparently beneficial effects of lytic phages at the population level.

The seasonality of cholera epidemics is worth a closer look. In Bangladesh, phages parasitizing cholera fluctuate seasonally as well. These fluctuations seem to track the density of cholera in a pattern that is well known to ecologists as the pattern of regular (animal–animal or animal–plant) predator–prey systems: the prey (cholera) increase first, then predators (phage) increase, causing prey to decrease once again. Once prey decrease, the predator of course decreases as well, having nothing to eat, allowing prey to increase once again and creating cycles of abundance. Thus, rather than the phage controlling the abundance of their prey, *V. cholerae*, the prey might well drive the abundance of the predator. Support for this idea comes from the observation that cholera epidemics in Haiti also show seasonality, but there doesn't seem to be any phage in the environment. Thus, either seasonality is driven by different mechanisms in the two locations, or the phage seasonality is a consequence rather than a cause of bacterial seasonality.

Contrary to what one might expect of an organism transmitted through drinking water, cholera thrives in salt water. It can also persist in fresh water, if the water is warm enough and contains enough nutrients. Epidemics in Bangladesh closely track surface sea water temperatures, for two reasons. First, warm sea surface water temperatures are associated with severe storms, which in turn cause flooding. Flooding worsens existing sanitation problems, co-mingling drinking water and sewage, and facilitating transmission of cholera.

Second, warm sea surface temperatures (particularly in association with large amounts of nutrients) cause blooms of tiny plants called phytoplankton. The phytoplankton are food for zooplankton—tiny floating marine animals. Cholera can stick to the exoskeletons of shrimp-like zooplankton known as copepods, whose bodies are made of a substance called chitin. Remember that a person needs to swallow huge numbers of cholera bacteria in order for any of them to survive our stomach acid. An individual copepod can accumulate ten thousand cholera bacteria: swallowing such a copepod is like ingesting a cholera bomb. If one such copepod arrives on a stomach full of food, enough cholera can easily be delivered to cause disease, while swallowing water with just a few free-living bacteria is unlikely to harm anyone. The ability of large numbers of cholera to stick to copepods has been used to explain how cholera outbreaks could arise from environmental sources of cholera, rather than from infected patients.

As with most other areas of science that matter at all, some parts of the cholera story are well accepted by the scientific community, while other parts are not. For example, scientists have long been puzzled by the fact that cholera behaves differently depending on the conditions under which it was reared. Cholera reared in laboratory culture is the standard on which estimates of the infectious dose (the number of particles required to make a person ill) are generally calculated. However, as lab-reared cholera fed to a volunteer go through the process of infecting the gut and being expelled in diarrhoea, these same bacteria can change to a *hyperinfectious* state. Far fewer numbers of these hyperinfectious bacteria are required to infect a new host. Without invoking such a hyperinfectious state, it's hard to explain how cholera can spread through a population so incredibly quickly—for example, there were 30,000 cases in just the first week of the 1991 cholera epidemic in Peru.

If hyperinfectious cholera reaches another human gut, it remains in the hyperinfectious state (as long as it doesn't get killed by lytic phage or hit with antibiotics). On the other hand, if it leaves a patient's bowels, enters the water, and fails to get taken up by another human victim for five to twenty-four hours, it undergoes another fundamental physiological change to a very different state called either 'viable but non-culturable' or 'active but non-culturable'. You can already see the controversy: even though this phenomenon has been known for more than thirty years, we can't even agree on what to call it! The non-culturable form of cholera has gained attention as a potential environmental reservoir for new cholera outbreaks. However, it's unknown whether or not this process is reversible, in particular, whether or not the bacteria can recover their ability to colonize humans after entering the non-culturable state.

An alternative environmental reservoir for cholera could come from the *persister* phenotype assumed by some cells after they enter water. When *V. cholerae* is starved for nutrients, as happens when it leaves the human gut and enters a water supply, some cells can enter this persistent state. Like the non-culturable states, the persistent state seems to involve dormancy, and involves changes in gene expression and morphology. However, persister bacteria *can* be cultured, and have been demonstrated experimentally to reawaken when provided with sufficient resources, particularly chitin.

One example of the importance of understanding sources of cholera outbreaks and the virulence of genes themselves comes from the ongoing cholera epidemic in Haiti. The tragedy of the 2010 earthquake in Haiti was heightened by an outbreak of cholera, with over 470,000 cases reported and 6,631 people dead in the first year. Haiti had been free of cholera cases for at least one hundred years, which raised the immediate question of how the disease had arrived. Analyses ranging from serotyping, to simple comparison of presence and absence of particular genes, to sophisticated phylogenetic analyses, have all suggested that the strains did not come from a local environmental source, such as the Gulf of Mexico.

Instead, the strains isolated from Haitian patients were most similar to strains from South East Asia, suggesting that they may have arrived with people from this area, or people who recently visited there—in this case, UN peacekeepers from Nepal. In addition, the camp of the peacekeepers was located on a tributary of the Artibonite River, which was identified as the source of the Haitian outbreak, although cholera rapidly spread throughout the country.

Chapter 6
Malaria

Malaria might be the most important infectious disease on the planet. Compared to the infectious diseases discussed in the previous chapters, it is less frightening to people in temperate, developed countries—not because it is less infectious or less virulent, but because in modern times it rarely reaches out of the tropics, being limited by the ecological niche of its mosquito vectors. Unlike cholera, malaria tends to be *endemic*—maintaining a relatively constant level in the population over time—rather than occurring in intense epidemic outbreaks. Typical of endemic disease, the most widespread strains of malaria are typically chronic and debilitating, rather than causing acute infection and death. The exception is falciparum malaria, most common in tropical sub-Saharan Africa. The malnutrition and anaemia associated with chronic malaria are associated with poorer educational outcomes in children, while acute malaria can lead to chronic neurological problems. Combining these non-lethal effects common to all malaria species with the lethal effects of falciparum, the cumulative impact of malaria on humanity is enormous.

Public health officials measure the impact of chronic diseases in terms of *disability-adjusted life years* (DALYs), which take into account both the loss of life and the loss of productivity and happiness due to a disease. Coming up with appropriate weights poses obvious ethical challenges. Is one year of life with a chronic, crippling disease equivalent to six months of healthy life? Three months? One month? How should one compare the impact of death or disability in an infant, a middle-aged person, or an elderly person? Nevertheless, DALY calculations account for the fact that the chronic effects of disease on people living with disease can be just as important, if not more important, than disease-induced deaths. In 2010, malaria accounted for more lost DALYs than any other infectious disease, narrowly edging out HIV/AIDS. Although hard evidence is difficult to come by—poor countries tend to be malarial while rich ones do not—researchers have suggested that eliminating malaria could increase economic growth rates by several percentage points, the difference between a struggling economy and a healthy one.

Although every infectious disease has its bizarre and intriguing quirks, malaria is more complex than the other diseases we have discussed so far. It is caused by a protozoan, a single-celled organism whose genetic material (unlike in bacteria) is confined within a nucleus. Its genome comprises about twenty-three million base pairs of DNA, thousands of times larger than the viral genomes of HIV and influenza and about five times larger than cholera's genome.

Malaria's complexity also stems from its *vector-borne* nature; it is transmitted from one human to another via various species of *Anopheles* mosquitoes. Cholera adjusts its biochemistry to function alternately as a free-living organism in the ocean and as a pathogen in the human gut. Malaria has an even more challenging problem; it adjusts its biochemistry to two different biological environments (the human host and mosquito vector), and to multiple organs within each host (human blood and liver; mosquito gut and salivary glands). Biological environments represent bigger challenges for parasitic organisms than physical environments. Desiccation and ultraviolet light are dangerous threats to parasites travelling through the physical environment outside the host, but they are passive. In contrast, host organisms take active steps to destroy parasitic hitchhikers by attacking them with immune defences.

Four species of malaria commonly infect humans. In order of decreasing severity, the malaria species are *Plasmodium falciparum*, *P. vivax*, *P. ovale*, and *P. malariae*. (Malaria species are referred to by the genus name *Plasmodium*, which can be abbreviated as *P.*, and their species name.) A fifth species, *P. knowlesi*, known originally as a disease of macaques, is emerging as a disease of humans in South East Asia, but so far only monkey-to-human (via mosquito) transmission, not human-to-human transmission, has been observed.

All malaria species have essentially the same life cycle. It starts with sexual reproduction (fusion of female and male *gametocytes*, the equivalent of eggs and sperm coming together) in the gut of a mosquito host, after which the next life stage (*sporozoites*) migrate to the mosquito salivary glands and are injected into the human host when the mosquito bites to get protein to feed her eggs. (Only mature female mosquitoes bite humans, which has important implications for malaria control.) The injected sporozoites migrate to the human's liver where they reproduce by simple division, migrate back to the bloodstream, and continue to multiply, infecting and destroying red blood cells as the population grows. Eventually the blood stages develop into female and male gametocytes and wait for another female mosquito to arrive and suck them up.

Malaria causes anaemia by destroying red blood cells. However, the worst symptoms occur when malaria parasites (most often *P. falciparum*) get into the brain, causing cerebral malaria. In cerebral malaria, parasites block blood flow and trigger inflammation, killing untreated patients and often causing brain damage even in patients who are treated and recover.

Malaria's most obvious symptom is fever, although fever does not itself seem to be harmful. Malarial fever recurs with characteristic frequency as new waves of parasites emerge from the liver into the blood: historically malaria strains were classified according to whether fever recurred every other day (*tertian*: *P. vivax* and *P. ovale*) or every three days (*quartan*: *P. malariae* and *P. falciparum*). In many malarial regions, patients who come to the hospital with fever and headache are automatically treated for malaria since testing is expensive and requires expertise.

Malaria's inability to move directly from one human to another opens up a wide range of possibilities for control. As Chapter 2 describes, Ronald Ross, one of the founders of disease modelling, figured out two important facts about malaria. First, he discovered that mosquitoes transmit malaria, which made it possible for the first time to prevent malaria by controlling mosquitoes, or by preventing them from biting humans (closing the encounter filter). Second, his models showed that public health agencies didn't need to completely eradicate mosquitoes to eradicate malaria—they just needed to reduce the number of mosquito bites by killing or repelling mosquitoes, until, on average, each malaria-infected person is bitten by so few mosquitoes that they lead to fewer than one new infection. The encounter filter doesn't need to be completely shut—just closed tightly enough that only a few mosquitoes can sneak through.

If you can't close the encounter filter by killing, blocking, or repelling mosquitoes in any of their life stages, you can try to close the compatibility filter. In prehistoric times, humans evolved many genetic mechanisms for closing the compatibility filter, although usually at a cost. Even before humans knew the cause of malaria, we developed drugs to block the compatibility filter by poisoning malaria within our bodies in ways that are somewhat less toxic to humans than to malaria. For example, gin and tonic was the favoured drink of British colonists in the tropics from the early 1800s on, due to the antimalarial action of the quinine found in tonic water. Most recently, we have tried to come up with vaccines to bolster our natural immunity, although so far without complete success. In what follows we will discuss all three of these compatibility-blocking strategies.

Biologists have retrieved ancient DNA from 4,000-year-old Egyptian mummies, but we know malaria is far older. Early relatives of malaria have been found in the guts of midges (biting flies) in amber, which were probably biting cold-blooded reptiles, from one hundred million years ago. However, such fossils are extremely rare, and in order to resolve the gap between one hundred million and 3,000 years ago we have to turn to the genome of malaria, and of its hosts.

Malaria parasites are part of a large, complex family, the apicomplexans, that frequently jump between hosts. Although the malaria parasites of lizards, birds, and mammals are all called *Plasmodium*, they are most likely two separate families (one that infects lizards and birds and one that infects mammals) that are more closely related to other parasites than to each other; mammalian malaria split off from the rest of the family around thirteen million years ago. The malaria species that infect humans are a similarly mixed group; they are all more closely related to various malaria parasites of non-human hosts than to each other, having split off somewhere around two to seven million years ago.

Exactly which non-human host various human malaria species jumped from, and when, is a rapidly developing and controversial story. Analyses of the genome of *P. falciparum*, the most dangerous species of human malaria, suggest that its population expanded greatly about 10,000 years ago, simultaneously with the development of agriculture and a concomitant increase in human population density. Where falciparum came from in the first place is a tougher question. While it is closely related to the chimpanzee malaria *P. reichenowi*, leading older textbooks to state that it jumped from chimpanzees into humans, two recent studies have made novel and contradictory claims. The first found more closely related malaria strains in blood samples from captive bonobos (a close relative of chimpanzees and humans); the second found more closely related strains in wild gorilla faeces. These results are still controversial; the authors of the gorilla study point out that falciparum-related infections are rare in wild chimpanzees and bonobos, and that therefore the bonobo infections are most likely to originate from humans. Regardless of our conclusions about falciparum's true origins, this tells us how tiny a window we still have into the complex ecosystem of malaria, its hosts, and their vectors.

The human genome sheds more light on the history of human–malaria interactions. Humans are not passive nurseries for malaria parasites; our immune systems are constantly evolving new ways to counter the parasite's debilitating effects. Humans have a variety of genetic anti-malaria strategies, with varying efficacy and severity of side effects. The best-known of these strategies is the sickle-cell trait, which appears in biology textbooks as an example of heterozygote advantage: individuals with one copy of the sickle-cell allele and one normal haemoglobin allele are partially tolerant of falciparum malaria, but having two copies of the allele causes crippling anaemia.

Thalassemia is another mutation similar to sickle-cell, relatively common in Mediterranean populations, that modifies red blood cells to reduce the severity of malarial symptoms at the price of anaemia. Glucose-6-phosphate-dehydrogenase (G6PD) deficiency, also common in Mediterranean populations, protects against falciparum and vivax malaria. G6PD also causes anaemia, but only under particular circumstances such as eating fava beans or taking common antimalarial drugs such as chloroquine or primaquine. Duffy negativity—the absence of the 'Duffy antigen', a protein that *P. vivax* and *P. knowlesi* target to enter red blood cells—prevents against malaria symptoms at the cost of a wide range of side effects.

Genetic analysis can estimate how long ago mutations arose. The well-known human blood type O appears to provide some protection from malaria, but it is so old—it has been around for millions of years, longer than human malaria itself—that it must originally have evolved for some reason other than malaria protection, probably to protect against some other now-unknown blood pathogen. Some variants of Duffy negativity are around 30,000 years old. G6PD deficiency arose 5,000 to 10,000 years ago, reinforcing the evidence from the falciparum genome that the risk to humans from falciparum malaria exploded around the time that agriculture developed. In contrast some sickle-cell variants are evolutionarily young—only a few hundreds or thousands of years old—reminding us that the human and malaria genomes are constantly (co)evolving.

Because these genetic protective mechanisms come with severe side effects, natural selection increases their frequencies only in regions where the risk of malaria outweighs the side effects. Elsewhere, it reduces their frequencies. Since malaria is so widespread and can have such deadly effects, it may be one of the strongest selective forces shaping the human genome in the past few thousand years. The geographic distributions of particular malaria-related genes (the Duffy antigen and sickle-cell in sub-Saharan Africa, thalassemia and G6PD deficiency around the Mediterranean) give evidence about the historical distribution of malaria. Because the side effects of malaria-protective genes are only one of the vast number of factors affecting human fitness, however, the stories told by human genetics and pathogen genes are sometimes complex. For example, researchers have traditionally assumed that the absence of the Duffy antigen in sub-Saharan Africa indicates that *P. vivax* originated there. Studies of the *P. vivax* genome complicated the story by linking vivax most closely to macaque (monkey) malarias from South East Asia, suggesting that Duffy negativity might have arisen for protection against other species of malaria or other malaria-like parasites, or after vivax made its way from Asia into Africa. Most recently, however, malaria DNA found in samples of wild gorilla faeces has again shifted the evidence back in favour of an African origin for vivax.

In addition to humans' evolved constitutive defences against malaria (systems that are in place whether or not a person has ever been infected), humans' adaptive immune systems can also help. Unfortunately, unlike the immune response to simple, acute viral diseases like measles, where immunity develops quickly and is essentially lifelong, malaria immunity develops slowly. No one completely understands why, although the huge variation in molecular markers among strains of malaria, and the ability of a single clone of malaria to switch its molecular appearance, is thought to be responsible. In high-malaria areas, people typically become tolerant to malaria as children, after they have already been infected several times. Malaria immunity generally wears off quickly, perhaps in part through the malaria parasite's interference with the human immune system.

Another problem is that humans' adaptive immunity to malaria provides more tolerance (also called *clinical immunity*) than resistance. In other words, immunity does reduce the number of parasites in the bloodstream, but its main effect is to reduce the severity of symptoms. This tolerance has two important implications: (1) people in high-malaria zones with clinical immunity won't feel sick, so they won't get treated even when treatments are available—this makes it harder to reduce malaria rates from high levels; (2) it will be correspondingly easier to keep malaria rates in check once malaria rates, and levels of clinical immunity, have been reduced.

For most of history, most humans have dealt with malaria by avoiding malarial zones (if they had a choice) or by living with it, hoping for some degree of attenuation of the symptoms through natural immunity. Our historical knowledge of malaria begins with humans' first attempts to consciously defend themselves against malaria. Humans discovered compatibility-blocking chemical defences against malaria long before they discovered the microorganisms that cause it. Jesuit priests brought the traditional medication quinine, derived from tree bark, to Europe in the early 17th century. Because South American natives chewed on the bark of the cinchona tree to stop shivering, the Jesuits guessed it might work on malarial fevers, which are often accompanied by shivering. The Jesuits got lucky; quinine doesn't actually reduce fever, but it does cure malaria by leading to the build up of toxic chemicals within blood-inhabiting stages of the malaria parasite.

While quinine can cure malaria, it is too expensive and too toxic to give it to everyone in the population regardless of whether they have malaria or not. Whenever possible, it's cheaper and safer to prevent disease by closing the encounter filter to block transmission rather than trying to close the compatibility filter once transmission has already happened. This idea applies to many diseases. Low-tech solutions like monogamy, or condoms, or clean needles, or hand sanitizer, or special water containers, work better (if you can get people to use them) than the best vaccines and treatments.

For malaria, the conclusion from this line of reasoning is that controlling malaria transmission (e.g. by covering water containers to remove suitable habitat for larval mosquitoes) may work better than treating people who are already infected. Sometimes mosquito reduction, and thus malaria control, occurs naturally as a side effect of changes in land use; changes in agricultural practice that reduced the amount of standing water available for mosquito breeding are thought to have led to declines in malaria in the northern US in the late 19th century. Of course, land use change can work in either direction. Abandonment of agricultural land in the southern US in the 1930s *increased* malaria infection. More recently, malaria in western Kenya has increased along with an increase in the number of active brick-making pits, which hold water but tend to have few mosquito-eating predators, providing a perfect habitat for larvae.

Prior to the discovery of DDT, public health authorities sometimes teamed up with engineers to reduce larval mosquito habitat by managing water—draining swamps or increasing water flow or changing water levels to make the habitat inhospitable to whatever local species of mosquito was transmitting malaria. They also sprayed oil or arsenic-based insecticides in the water to kill larvae. In a form of biological control, health authorities introduced larvae-eating fish, especially the genus *Gambusia*, which is called the mosquitofish due to its dietary habits. In the first half of the 20th century, mosquitofish were brought from North America to malarial regions all over the world, from South America to central Asia to Italy to Palestine. However, it's hard to know exactly how well they worked since they were usually combined with other control measures such as water management and chemical spraying.

While such forms of source reduction were somewhat effective in developed countries, temperate or semi-arid regions, and other areas where malaria spread slowly, they were often impractical for poor, humid, tropical countries where malaria was rampant. Paul Hermann Müller's discovery of the insecticidal properties of DDT in 1939, for which he won the Nobel Prize in 1948, revolutionized malaria control. It triggered a shift from environmental and ecological engineering focused on destroying mosquitoes in their larval habitats, to protection by killing adult mosquitoes in the vicinity of humans. Indoor residual spraying programmes apply long-lasting insecticide to surfaces in houses where mosquitoes like to land. They work extremely well if a cheap, long-lasting, relatively non-toxic (to humans) insecticide such as DDT is available. Houses may only need to be sprayed a few times a year, depending on the climate and the characteristics of the wall surfaces. In general, residual spraying works better than trying to exclude mosquitoes from houses—not only is it usually cheaper, but it kills mosquitoes rather than just excluding them, thus potentially providing some protection in the area around houses. Residual spraying programmes recorded initial successes all over the world: malaria was finally eliminated from the US in the early 1950s after decades of source reduction, while residual spraying (with DDT and with other insecticides) in many African countries significantly lowered the malaria burden, at least initially.

The second great post-war advance in malaria control was the development of chloroquine, a cheaper and relatively non-toxic biochemical variant of quinine. Chloroquine was first synthesized by German scientists after World War I. At that time the Allies controlled Java, which had most of the world's supply of quinine, depriving German troops in East Africa of this vital drug. During World War II, the tables turned when the Japanese took over Java; US researchers then developed chloroquine into an effective antimalarial, although again too late to help their soldiers (who were located this time in Sicily and South East Asia). The mass administration of chloroquine both improved individual health by curing sick people of malaria, and reduced the threat of malaria at the population level by reducing the chances that a malarial person would pass the pathogen on to a mosquito. In addition to its other advantages, chloroquine helps control the sexual stages of most malaria species, thus blocking transmission as well as helping the infected person.

The combined power of DDT and chloroquine, along with other synthetic insecticides and treatments, made global health agencies very optimistic in the 1950s that malaria could be controlled and even eradicated. However, malaria control efforts in the most resistant zones—rural districts of poor, tropical countries—ran into unanticipated problems after a few decades. Even though DDT and chloroquine were relatively cheap, non-toxic, and effective, the financial and logistical difficulties of mounting a global malaria campaign were greater than anyone had imagined.

First, like all campaigns to help people in less developed countries, malaria control programmes run into logistical, administrative, and cultural roadblocks. Does the local government actually send the supplies out to the places they're most needed? Do people steal them for other uses? Are the roads good enough to get them there? If they get there, can you train people to use them properly? Local residents may not want to use DDT, because it smells bad and stains their walls. They may resent foreign intrusion. Conflicts may break out and interrupt the programme, sending you back to square one. Funding agencies may tire of donating money after a few years, or they may decide that some other problem—feeding people, or providing them with clean water, or preventing a different disease such as Ebola—is more important.

The Global Malaria Eradication Program, which began in 1955 and aimed to eradicate malaria by 1963, encountered all of these problems, and more, before it was finally abandoned in 1969, although it did reduce the malaria mortality rate more than tenfold from its 1900 baseline. Another unforeseen problem with the campaign was the linkage of DDT use to bird deaths in North America publicized in Rachel Carson's *Silent Spring* (1962), leading to a ban on the pesticide within the US and later Canada.

Second, like all infectious disease control efforts, the enemies you're fighting are biological organisms, and they will evolve countermeasures against your control strategies. Resistance evolves both in malaria vectors (against DDT and other synthetic insecticides) and in the pathogen itself (against chloroquine and other synthetic antimalarial drugs). The basic principle of chemical control is to poison the target organism—introduce a chemical that disrupts some aspect of its physiology or biochemistry, without being too toxic to the host (for chemotherapeutic agents) or other species in the environment (for vector control agents). The target is then under very strong selection pressure to either (1) change its biology in a way that neutralizes the effects of the chemical, or (2) develop ways to detoxify the chemical or remove it from its cells.

Mosquitoes gain resistance to chloroquine by inheriting mutations that pump the chemical out of their cells. No one knows exactly when these mutations first occurred, but they spread very rapidly; chloroquine resistance in *P. falciparum* was first detected in the late 1950s in South America and South East Asia, and appeared in Africa in the 1970s. By the mid-2000s, chloroquine resistance had spread globally. Luckily, a new antimalarial drug called artemisinin, rediscovered by Chinese researchers screening historically known cures for fever, was available at that time. Artemisinin is now the first-line drug of choice for malaria treatment; however, it, too, has already seen the evolution of partial resistance so far contained to South East Asia. The World Health Organization is actively trying to prevent resistance from spreading, primarily by making sure that artemisinin is always used in combination with other antimalarial drugs to radically decrease the probability that strains of malaria will be able to evolve to resist both drugs simultaneously, much in the same way that resistance to HAART treatment for HIV is extremely rare because three drugs are used.

DDT-resistant mosquitoes have genetic modifications that either change the biochemistry of their neurons (the target of DDT), or allow them to detoxify DDT within their bodies. DDT resistance had already begun to be detected by the mid-1950s, and is widespread today, although levels of resistance vary enormously from country to country and from one mosquito species to another. Some researchers argue that DDT resistance comes in large part from heavy agricultural use (against insects other than mosquitoes, but exposing mosquitoes as a by-product), and that DDT could have been much more effective if had been restricted to use in disease control programmes. While in principle mosquito populations could also lose DDT resistance if managers stopped using DDT in an area, experiments in flies have shown that DDT resistance seems to carry little if any fitness cost, so that DDT resistance is likely to persist for a long time. Malaria control programmes now try to manage resistance by switching among a variety of different synthetic insecticides that vary in their cost, effectiveness against mosquitoes, and toxicity to humans or other insects or wildlife.

In the last few decades international efforts towards malaria eradication and control have ramped up again. Planners have learned lessons from the failures of earlier programmes: in particular, they are more aware of the importance of political and cultural context, of using different strategies in different regions, and of considering malaria control programmes as part of a more general improvement in health infrastructure. They have also scaled back their optimism about eradication: the new international programme is called the Global Malaria *Action* (rather than 'Eradication') Plan (GMAP), and aims only for local elimination from particular countries. While GMAP does state that spending on malaria control can decrease as malaria is eliminated from some countries, so that money only needs to be spent making sure that it stays eliminated, current spending rates are about US$2.5 billion per year out of the US$8–10 billion that might be necessary for control and eradication—and this level of commitment will probably need to be maintained for decades.

Current efforts to control malaria have one new tool that was not available in the 1960s—insecticide-treated bed nets (ITNs) using pyrethroids, a class of insecticide that is safe for mammals (although toxic to fish). Pyrethroid-based ITNs were first deployed in the 1980s; long-lasting versions that can kill mosquitoes for five years beyond the six months' effectiveness of the original ITNs were deployed in the early 2000s. The idea of ITNs is not that different from indoor residual spraying—they kill mosquitoes that come indoors to bite humans—but they have the additional advantages of providing a physical as well as a chemical barrier, and working even in houses that have porous walls unsuitable for spraying. They have their logistical and cultural problems—for example, recipients have been known to use the nets for catching or drying fish rather than for malaria protection. However, given that no malaria control strategy is 100 per cent effective by itself, ITNs provide a vital addition to the malaria control arsenal.

One lesson of bed nets is that a long-lasting tool is nearly always better—more cost-effective and requiring less effort to deliver—than its short-lived counterpart. A bed net that needs to be replaced every five years is better, all other things equal, than a residual spraying programme that needs to be repeated every six months, even though the bed net only works when people sleep under it. A malaria vaccine, even if an imperfect and short-lived one, would be the compatibility filter analogue of bed nets; rather than treating people with artemisinin only after they got sick, you could just vaccinate them every few years. No malaria vaccine is yet (as of January 2015) available for use, but the currently most promising vaccine, which protected 25–50 per cent of children in clinical trials, is scheduled for use within the next few years. Researchers think it will be more cost-effective than bed nets in some areas.

We are still deeply ignorant about malarial parasites. Knowing more about the ancient history of different malaria strains—when, and from where, they entered the human population—would deepen our understanding of the zoonotic processes that give rise to new human strains. Knowing more about the current distribution and ecology of malaria in non-human primates could help us guess about the likelihood of future zoonotics. Increased sampling of wild populations, and faster and cheaper genomic scans of malaria and primate genomes, are helping to resolve the picture, but it is anyone's guess how completely we will ever understand either the ecology or the evolutionary history of malaria.

So what does the future hold for malaria control? There is some room for optimism. In the absence of major economic or political shocks to the developing world, or the emergence or re-emergence of pathogens that shift the focus away from malaria, the current efforts of many countries and foundations will continue to chip away at the burden of malaria over the next few decades. Elimination is possible in many areas, but malaria experts are at best cautiously optimistic about eradication.

Along with the evolution of mosquitoes and malaria, climate change and (more importantly) land use and economic change will continually move the target. No single magic bullet will solve the problem of malaria. Governments and agencies will have to deploy different combinations of the available tools (source control, residual spraying, bed nets, treatment, and eventually vaccine) in ways that are appropriate to the local situation.

Chapter 7 *Batrachochytrium dendrobatidis*

Batrachochytrium dendrobatidis (Bd), the subject of our last case study, differs in many ways from the earlier examples. This fungus is the first (and only) non-human pathogen we will discuss. Its genome is many times larger than the viruses and bacteria considered earlier, similar in size to the malaria protozoan's. It is a generalist pathogen, infecting hundreds of different amphibian species and driving some of them to extinction.

Most important, Bd is our first example of an *emerging* pathogen. In practice, the definition of an emerging pathogen is very broad; it essentially means a pathogen that we are newly concerned about for some reason. The pathogen may be truly novel, emerging through mutation. More commonly, zoonotic pathogens emerge when existing pathogens jump to a new species. We may also classify disease as emerging when we detect a previously known pathogen in a known host, but in a new geographic region. Alternatively, emergence might describe an increase in the virulence or transmission of an existing pathogen (due to mutation, or to some change in the host or the environment). Finally, hosts might have become less tolerant or less resistant due to a genetic or environmental change.

For emerging pathogens of humans, the prime suspect is zoonosis (as in HIV), sometimes combined with pathogen mutation (as in pandemic influenza). Human pathogens can also emerge when environmental change opens the environmental filter for an existing disease, as when mosquito vectors of dengue spread to North America, or when people increased their contact with Lyme-disease-bearing ticks by building houses in wooded areas.

Emerging diseases of non-human species are a concern for several reasons. Many non-human species are economically valuable; emerging disease can threaten our wallets or even our lives. Agricultural disease can threaten important crops. The Irish potato blight—a fungal pathogen that jumped from its origin in South America to Europe via North America—caused massive human mortality and fundamentally altered the history of Ireland.

Diseases can also affect economically important wild populations. The recent decline in honeybees, the causes of which are still hotly debated but are due in part to pathogen spread, has severely compromised the California almond crops they pollinate; chronic wasting disease in wild elk threatens to cost Canadian elk farmers millions of dollars. Hopefully, we would also care about the welfare of non-human organisms for selfless reasons—conserving non-human species is simply the right thing to do.

Bd in amphibians is definitely in the latter category—despite the economic value of some amphibian species in the frog-leg trade or in controlling pests, most of the species affected by Bd are economically unimportant. Nevertheless, we want to understand where Bd came from and discover how we can protect wild amphibian populations from its impact. The concepts and strategies we use in our efforts to determine Bd's origin can also serve as a case study for understanding and controlling future emerging diseases of non-human species.

Physiology and natural history

Bd is the black sheep of a large and otherwise mostly obscure family of fungi, the chytrids. While a few chytrid fungi attack other fungi or plants, most live harmlessly on decaying organic matter in aquatic environments. Bd is one of only two known chytrids that attacks vertebrates, the second being a salamander pathogen that was only discovered in 2013. (Chytrid biologists complain when people refer to Bd as '*the* chytrid fungus', feeling that this unfairly taints all chytrids with the misbehaviour of one species.) Bd lives on and within the skin of amphibians, especially on keratin, a hard protein found in the skin. Its life cycle alternates between structures called *thalli*—bottle-shaped cells that grow within the host's skin layers—and *zoospores*, small mobile cells that disperse from the thalli into the water, eventually landing either back on the same host's skin or on another host, thus spreading the infection.

We know very little about when and how Bd persists in the environment, away from its host organisms. This is a critical question if we want to understand how Bd spreads from one amphibian population to another; whether populations can recover or recolonize years after they have been locally extirpated by Bd; and how to design quarantine programmes to protect healthy populations from Bd. Given that many of Bd's relatives are free-living microbes, it would not be surprising if Bd also retained the capability to survive and grow in the environment. We know that Bd can persist in pure water for weeks or months, and thrives on the keratin found in amphibian skins, feathers, and the exoskeletons of insects and crustaceans such as shrimp and crayfish. At present, however, we don't know if Bd can persist for years, or move long distances, in the absence of a host.

Bd might persist between seasons on tadpoles. This life stage is more tolerant because tadpoles only have keratin around their mouths, which they may be able to discard in response to infection without dying. This form of *intraspecific reservoir*, where pathogens persist in a tolerant life stage of the same species, has also been suggested for other amphibian pathogens. Many kinds of tadpoles grow slower but don't die when infected with Bd; in other species tadpoles do die from Bd. The most important reservoirs and vectors of Bd infection are probably individuals from tolerant host species, which can harbour the fungi and pass them to new (or recovering) populations without being harmed themselves. Most amphibian communities contain tolerant hosts—researchers are still trying to understand what makes a host tolerant or intolerant of Bd. Some of the most important potential players are some species of crayfish, the American bullfrog, and the South African clawed frog *Xenopus laevis*. All of these species are widespread, have been able to invade new geographic regions with or without human help, and are tolerant of at least some strains of Bd.

Another item on the long list of things we don't know about Bd is how it kills its hosts. Researchers have speculated about various causes, including the production by Bd of some kind of toxin. However, most of the current evidence suggests that infected adult frogs typically die when the build up of Bd in their skin and its subsequent thickening and hardening prevents them from maintaining proper salt concentrations in their bodies, leading to death by cardiac arrest.

Amphibian species vary wildly in their susceptibility to Bd: wide variation in space, time, across species, and across communities is a hallmark of this emerging disease. Some of this variation may stem from differences in host defence. The immune systems of *Xenopus* frogs produce antibodies that recognize Bd, although there is only weak evidence at present that these proteins protect against the fungus. The evidence is stronger for the protective effect of the antimicrobial proteins that many species of frogs and toads secrete on to their skins; species whose skin secretions inhibit Bd in a test tube also tend to survive infection better.

Finally, some species seem to have the capacity to generate behavioural 'fevers' in response to Bd, which grows fastest between seventeen and twenty-three degrees Celsius, but dies at temperatures of thirty degrees Celsius and higher. Although frogs are cold-blooded and can't shiver to raise their body temperatures, infected frogs can and do boost their body temperatures by spending more time in warm, sunny places, which appears to help them recover from Bd. Frogs can even be cured of Bd in the lab by putting them in warm environments for less than a day. Not all species can be cured in this way, suggesting that rather than harming Bd directly, warm temperatures may help frogs by improving their ability to produce antimicrobial proteins. Some of the variation among species could also be explained by the fact that different species are tested by different researchers, in different labs, using different experimental procedures.

Discovery

Ecologists discovered Bd in the late 1990s when frogs throughout eastern Australia and Central America started dying from mysterious causes. At about the same time, poison dart frogs in the US National Zoo also started dying. Veterinary researchers there got in touch with the few researchers in the world who knew anything about this previously obscure family of fungi. Between them they came up with a species description and a name based on the Latin name of poison dart frogs, *Dendrobates*: the genus name *Batrachochytrium* means 'chytrid that infects frogs and toads'.

One interesting sidelight of the discovery of Bd is the experience of Joyce Longcore, an expert on chytrid fungi. After keeping house and raising children for twenty years, Longcore went back to graduate school, receiving a PhD in mycology in 1991. As of 1997, just before the discovery of Bd, she looked set for a quiet career studying an obscure family of fungi. When Bd suddenly exploded in importance, she was the go-to person for information about the biology of chytrid fungi, and her career took off like a rocket. Since 1998 she has co-authored sixty-four papers with more than 3,700 total citations, making her a scientific star. Her story demonstrates the value of having the right knowledge at the right time. It also shows that seemingly arcane biological knowledge can suddenly become vital to understand a novel ecological situation.

Once it became clear that Bd was a previously unknown pathogen, biologists asked about its origins: had it arrived recently in the communities it was destroying, or had it lain dormant in those communities for millennia before suddenly beginning to cause harm? The ensuing debate between the *novel pathogen hypothesis* (NPH) and the *endemic pathogen hypothesis* (EPH), versions of which apply to most emerging diseases of wildlife, has been raging ever since. Although we have generated a huge amount of information about Bd and its interaction with amphibians in the two decades since its discovery, the debate continues: it seems that every time a new piece of research supports the NPH, another study follows quickly to add evidence for the EPH.

The NPH does not say that Bd is a new species—we know that it existed long before the 1990s. Rather, it says that Bd, or at least virulent strains of Bd, is new to the specific geographic areas in which we now see infected populations. If the NPH is true, then Bd must have moved into new areas around the time when disease-related die-offs were first observed. Under the NPH we would expect to see a clear spatial separation between regions where Bd has and has not yet arrived, rather than a patchwork of local regions with and without Bd-related die-offs. We should also be able to see a signature of its rapid spread in the spatial pattern of its genes, with high genetic diversity in regions where it has persisted for a long time and low genetic diversity in areas with recent disease outbreaks.

In contrast, the EPH asserts that the same strains of Bd have been present in amphibian communities, even the ones that have undergone recent disease outbreaks, for a long time. The *disease triangle*, an idea from plant epidemiology, says that a disease outbreak requires the presence of (1) a suitable host, (2) a pathogen, and (3) an environment in which the pathogen can overcome the encounter and compatibility filters in order to successfully spread from one host to another, and overcome tolerance to cause disease. The EPH says that the first two sides of the triangle have been in place for centuries or millennia, but that some change in the environment has recently opened the encounter and compatibility filters, or changed tolerance. Since Bd must (as far as we know now) be able to infect amphibian hosts in order to persist in the long term, it is not the encounter (transmission) or compatibility (resistance) filter that has opened; rather, proponents of the EPH think that changes in the environment have made hosts less tolerant of Bd, or equivalently have made Bd more virulent. To validate the EPH, we should not only fail to validate the predictions of the NPH (both the spatial distribution of Bd and its spatial pattern of genetic variation should be noisy and unpredictable); we should also be able to identify environmental covariates that predict whether hosts are tolerant/Bd is virulent in a particular community, and we should be able to find evidence that these covariates have changed recently in outbreak regions.

Before we go through the evidence for each hypothesis, it's worth keeping in mind that Bd emergence is complex—like all biological phenomena—and that the NPH and EPH are not mutually exclusive. It could be true both that Bd has recently moved into new geographic regions (as stated by the NPH), *and* that Bd has become more virulent or hosts have lost tolerance (as stated by the EPH).

We start with the historical and genetic evidence, which should help us determine when Bd arrived in different locations around the globe. As is the case with nearly all infectious diseases of wildlife, Bd existed long before biologists noticed it in amphibian communities. Unlike human diseases such as malaria or influenza, however, there are no historical records that can tell us where Bd was in the past—even if there had been ancient plagues where frogs and toads started dying in huge numbers, humans probably wouldn't have noticed. In fact, even when people *did* notice amphibian die-offs in the recent past, such as the disappearance of boreal toads from the mountains of Colorado in the 1970s, or the decline of *Atelopus* frogs in Central America in the late 1980s—declines that we attribute retrospectively to Bd—they attributed them to other causes, such as climate change or environmental stress coupled with bacterial outbreaks.

With the advent of good methods for identifying DNA—similar to those used in the archaeological discoveries of malaria in Egyptian mummies—researchers are able to go back in time by trying to detect Bd DNA on the skins of frogs borrowed from the collections of natural history museums. In both Colorado and Central America, they successfully recovered chytrid fungi from frog skins collected around the time of the outbreaks, making Bd-induced die-offs extremely plausible in hindsight. However, these results do not strongly support either the NPH or the EPH, since the researchers have not been able to show the *absence* of Bd in those areas in periods just before the outbreaks.

Researchers were excited to discover Bd DNA on the skins of *Xenopus* collected in South Africa in 1938. The early appearance of Bd associated with this widespread, tolerant species led them to propose the 'Out of Africa' hypothesis—the idea that the strains of Bd that would later originate the global Bd pandemic evolved in Africa some time prior to 1938 and only began to spread globally after a human pregnancy test based on *Xenopus* eggs was developed in the 1930s, leading to the export of thousands of *Xenopus* a year from South Africa. According to this hypothesis, the fungus would have had two decades to spread globally during the 1940s and 1950s (before other pregnancy tests replaced the *Xenopus*-egg test), after which it gradually spread in new habitats, perhaps via other tolerant hosts.

However, these hypotheses are fragile—every time someone sets a new record by discovering Bd on an even older preserved amphibian skin, the story changes. Twin discoveries in 2013 and 2014 drastically shifted the grounds of the debate. First, researchers detected Bd on the skin of a bullfrog collected in 1928, in California. Bullfrogs had previously been suspected of spreading Bd across amphibian communities. This finding did not completely rule out the Out of Africa hypothesis, but it complicated it considerably. Since the Bd finding in California is too early for the pregnancy-test-driven export of *Xenopus* from Africa, either Bd would have to have jumped out of Africa more than ten years earlier via some other process, or the strain of Bd found in the Californian frog skin would have to represent a different (non-virulent) lineage. Next, in an even more sensational finding, a group of researchers discovered Bd on a quarter of the frogs from a huge collection from the Atlantic forest of Brazil going all the way back to 1894.

While researchers will keep pushing back these records, finding earlier and earlier occurrences of Bd around the globe, new discoveries get progressively harder as we go back in time simply because we have fewer museum specimens to test. Turning instead to the evidence from Bd's genome, we find again—as with so many aspects of Bd—that it's complicated. There are many families (lineages) of Bd, of which the most important (from our point of view) is the so-called *global pandemic lineage* (GPL), which contains all of the samples collected from amphibian populations that are in decline and a few others. In the first phylogenetic studies of Bd, GPL appeared to have the exact characteristics of a rapidly spreading pathogen family: the very low level of genetic variation among its members and lack of recognizable geographic pattern could both be explained by a process where pathogens colonized new communities much faster than they could evolve new genotypes characteristic of a particular region. More recent studies have once again complicated the picture. While the GPL still appears geographically chaotic, containing representative Bd strains from every region, a growing database and more thorough genome scans have shown researchers that it also contains considerable variation; the newest studies have increased the estimated age of the most recent ancestor of the GPL from as little as decades (consistent with an emerging pathogen that first arose around the time of *Xenopus* exports from Africa) to at least 10,000 years. Furthermore, the direct historical evidence from Brazilian frogs shows that, wherever the GPL originated, strains of Bd from that GPL lineage have been physically present in South America, apparently not leading to population declines and extinctions in amphibian communities, for a century.

We can hope that more analysis of museum skins, and still more thorough genome scans, may yet clarify the history of the lineages that are currently designated as the GPL. Deeper study may eventually succeed in dividing the GPL strains cleanly into one low-virulence group that has existed all over the world for millennia and a new, high-virulence group, possibly arising from hybridization between existing strains. As it spread from one geographic region to another over decades, this new group would have contributed to the retrospectively identified Bd-driven amphibian declines in Colorado in the 1970s, Central America in the 1980s, and eastern Australia and Central America in the 2000s.

On the other hand, the failure of the data to tell a compelling, uncomplicated story supporting the NPH may lead researchers back towards the EPH. In the early days—just after the discovery of the declines in Central America and Australia, and especially as it became obvious that the impact of Bd varied drastically from one community to another—researchers scrambled to find environmental changes that could explain the (apparently) sudden virulence of Bd. One of the puzzling aspects of Bd-induced die-offs was that they often seemed to occur in high-elevation, pristine areas such as nature reserves—inconsistent with a story involving human-induced changes to the landscape. Two environmental factors that researchers initially thought might be interacting with Bd to cause die-offs, by stressing amphibians or depressing their immune responses, were pesticide contamination (possibly blown long distances from agricultural areas) and ultraviolet radiation (consistent with effects of elevation). Despite some associations with population declines, and some lab studies that have shown that ultraviolet radiation and pesticides can make Bd more virulent, these factors have not (yet) provided much power for predicting where and when Bd will strike amphibian communities.

Temperature has a stronger signal: it has been consistently associated with harmful effects of Bd both on individual animals in lab studies and on communities in nature. As already mentioned, studies have consistently shown that Bd does best within a narrow thermal window. Temperature can potentially explain the pattern of high-elevation die-offs, since temperatures are consistently cooler at higher elevations. However, while it may explain why lowland communities persist while their uphill neighbours are being destroyed by disease, it doesn't explain the temporal patterns—why have high-elevation communities only begun to be destroyed in the last few decades and not before, if (as often seems to be the case) Bd has been present for centuries? What has changed?

The most obvious candidate, and one that is always on environmentalists' radar, is human-induced climate change. Perhaps climate change, which we know severely affects ecological communities at high latitudes and high altitudes, has recently shifted conditions past a tipping point that allows Bd to spread and/or harm communities, either by increasing the growth rate of Bd (e.g. the zoospore production rate) or by lowering the compatibility filter of individual amphibians.

The climate change hypothesis has been controversial within the Bd research community. A high-profile 2006 study suggested that reduced daily temperature variation in the Central American highlands had facilitated outbreaks by allowing Bd to remain in its optimal thermal range more of the time. Other researchers claimed that this study made mistakes about important details such as the lag between temperature changes, Bd outbreaks, and community die-offs. Furthermore, the spatio-temporal pattern of the die-offs—which spread across Central America at a rate of hundreds of kilometres per year rather than affecting the entire region simultaneously—seemed more characteristic of the spread of a novel pathogen than of a change in regional climate. In support of the original hypothesis, subsequent analyses using the same climate and die-off data as well as additional climatic measurements suggested that changes in temperature variability, rather than mean temperature, were indeed associated with the die-offs, even after taking the spatial pattern of spread into account, and that die-offs might have been driven by local effects of the global decade-scale climate shift called El Niño, rather than by longer-term human-induced climate change. A global study of Bd die-offs found that annual precipitation is correlated with die-offs, although other similar studies failed to find a strong effect. While changes in climate may well contribute to the occurrence and impact of Bd outbreaks, they do not provide the smoking gun that the proponents of the EPH are looking for.

As the Bd story gets ever more complex, many biologists acknowledge that neither the NPH nor the EPH is ever going to tell the whole story. Are we any closer to understanding when, where, and why Bd occurs, and where it has dire consequences for amphibian populations? Yes. While science sometimes seems to go in a circle—researchers are still focused on the same hypotheses that framed the initial debates when Bd was first discovered—closer examination often shows, more encouragingly, that the path is more like an ever-narrowing helix. We return to the same arguments, but at a higher level, with a new level of sophistication and drawing on new kinds of evidence. The extraction of Bd genomic data from recent and historical collections has given us a much deeper understanding of the distribution of Bd in space and time, and several new techniques promise more insights. Genomic data from amphibian hosts can provide evidence about past population bottlenecks; looking at the genes for antimicrobial proteins can suggest which species needed to defend themselves from Bd in the past. On the EPH side, proxies for past climate such as the isotopic composition of trees or soil (which reveal patterns of temperature and dryness) can give us a more complete picture of the way the host–pathogen–environment disease triangle worked in ancient environments.

Beyond intellectual satisfaction, does any of this information help us control Bd outbreaks or lessen their impact on amphibian communities? The NPH versus EPH debate has implications for Bd control strategies. If the NPH is correct, implying that the environment has *not* changed in important ways and that what's new is the presence of the pathogen, then conservationists should focus on preventing spread across communities. If the EPH is correct—i.e. the pathogen has been present all along but the environment has worsened—then we should worry about making the environment better for amphibians so that they can resist or tolerate Bd.

However, the dichotomy might be less practically useful than it first appears. *If* we can intervene to reverse the triggering change—the presence of the pathogen or the change in the environment—then we can protect amphibians. But it's not practical to remove Bd from the environment once it has arrived, and we can't change the occurrence of El Niño events or anthropogenic global change (at least not on a useful time scale). Conservation actions must be based on the overlap of actions that we think will attack the root causes of disease emergence, actions that are ethical (is it OK to cull some members of an endangered species to save the rest?), and actions that are logistically feasible.

Even without knowing anything about the disease, we can close the encounter filter by transporting individuals from the wild into disease-free, artificial habitats. The Amphibian Ark is a project that aims to preserve species by making sure that, no matter what happens in nature, we have some animals in captive breeding programmes that can (hopefully) be reintroduced into the wild once we have figured out how to control Bd. Biologists are already successfully rearing endangered species in captivity, but we don't know when or how we'll be able to reintroduce them. Captive rearing buys time, but eventually we either need to breed Bd-resistant variants of these species, or find a way to control Bd in nature. It also raises ethical issues: might we be harming endangered species by removing individuals from the wild? Could the existence of captive populations reduce the urgency we feel to deal with the problem? Is it OK to raise funds for conservation by raising additional captive animals for sale?

The next most direct way to try to save amphibians is by closing the compatibility filter for individuals in the wild. Antifungal drugs and temperature-raising treatments have worked to cure frogs of Bd in laboratory trials, and we may be able to scale these treatments up to capture, treat, and release enough individuals to save wild populations. Biologists have also proposed to treat amphibians with skin peptides from resistant species, or to treat individuals or even entire communities with a bacterium that produces antifungal compounds that suppress Bd. Very recently, researchers have discovered that exposing some amphibians to dead Bd in the lab can give them partial resistance to Bd, although it is too soon to know whether this finding can be used to develop a practical disease-fighting strategy.

The fight against Bd faces the same two fundamental problems as every other disease control and prevention programme—lack of knowledge and lack of resources. No matter how cute or interesting the victims are, diseases of wild animals will never command the same interest as human disease, so we will always have fewer resources—and less knowledge, since resources are needed to acquire knowledge. We do have some advantages—we can cull animals if it looks like it will help us to control an outbreak, breed animals for disease tolerance or resistance, and induce experimental infections to evaluate treatments (all strategies that would be looked on unfavourably for human pathogen control). Since we haven't yet managed to deploy any disease control strategies in the field, we haven't yet had to worry about evolutionary countermeasures taken by the pathogen, although these are bound to happen once we start to take action.

Although infectious diseases of wild animals differ from those of humans in superficial ways, the physiological, ecological, and evolutionary dynamics that drive them are very similar. In the long run, analysing wildlife disease helps us understand the fundamental properties of infectious disease. It can help protect harvested or hunted populations that are economically valuable. Understanding how disease moves in natural populations may also provide early-warning systems to detect zoonotic diseases that can jump into humans. Perhaps most fundamentally, many biologists (including the authors of this book) feel that we have an ethical responsibility to preserve species when we can, especially when our actions may have contributed to the spread of diseases that threaten them.

Chapter 8
Looking ahead

This book has given a whirlwind tour of some important infectious diseases, their ecological and evolutionary principles, and how these principles inform treatment and control. We chose a few case studies we could fit into the book on the basis of socio-economic importance and ecological/evolutionary interest, covering a broad range of disease-causing taxa. Our choice was admittedly biased towards diseases we thought would be familiar to our readers.

We have regretfully omitted many infectious diseases that hurt many people, costing hundreds of thousands of lives, millions of disability-adjusted life years, and billions of dollars. Some examples include tuberculosis (the most important disease we have neglected), polio, and schistosomiasis (a parasitic disease that causes liver damage, mostly affecting people in sub-Saharan Africa). So many such diseases are rampant in less developed tropical countries that there is an entire category, 'neglected tropical diseases', and a scientific journal devoted to them.

We have also left out fascinating diseases that have shaped history. The bubonic plague, the greatest infectious killer ever, is now relatively easy to treat with antibiotics. Smallpox, the first disease to be eradicated in the wild by vaccination, destroyed native populations in the Americas and was used to facilitate European colonization. Finally, rinderpest, a cattle disease closely related to measles, may have transformed the landscape of east Africa by wiping out native wildlife and allowing the growth of shrubby vegetation which allowed tsetse flies, and through them a vector-borne disease called sleeping sickness or trypanosomiasis, to establish.

For the most part, we have focused on established diseases rather than emerging diseases, although HIV and Bd have emerged relatively recently, and the 2009 pandemic H1N1 strain of influenza could count as 'recently emerged'. We haven't had room to discuss emerging coronaviruses such as SARS or MERS; the henipaviruses such as Nipah virus that threaten to spill over from fruit bats in Australia and South East Asia; or emergent vector-borne diseases such as West Nile and dengue viruses, or the bacteria causing Lyme disease.

Finally, we have covered only a small range of the kinds of organisms that can cause infectious disease. Admittedly, viruses such as influenza and HIV, bacteria such as *Vibrio cholerae*, protozoans such as the malarial agent *Plasmodium falciparum*, and fungi such as *Batrachochytrium dendrobatidis* make up the vast majority of pathogenic agents. However, we have passed over multicellular parasites such as roundworms (nematodes) and flatworms (platyhelminths), which have traditionally been thought of separately from microparasitic infectious diseases (see Chapter 2), but which are driven by the same epidemiological, ecological, and evolutionary principles. Multicellular parasites and protozoans make up the majority of neglected tropical diseases. The general restriction of these diseases to relatively poor, less-developed countries, as well as their tendency to cause chronic debility rather than acute disease, contribute to their traditional relegation to a separate category.

In the past few decades, researchers have also discovered several absolutely new modes of infectious disease that seem almost like science fiction. The first, *prions* or transmissible infectious proteins, are misfolded proteins that can replicate within a host by catalysing the misfolding of other proteins to the prion form. Prion diseases such as scrapie, known to infect sheep since the 1700s, and chronic wasting disease, which was first detected infecting deer in Colorado in the 1960s, are probably transmitted from one animal to another when animals eat vegetation contaminated with prion proteins. Prion proteins get on to plants, completing the transmission cycle, through environmental contamination from animals' bodily fluids (saliva, faeces, or amniotic fluids) or when released into the soil from their cadavers.

Prion diseases hit the headlines in the 1990s with 'mad cow disease', officially called bovine spongiform encephalopathy (the condition is drily called 'variant Creutzfeldt–Jakob disease' when it occurs in humans). Along with the fear of contracting a disease that leads to fatal neurological degeneration, the British public was also fascinated by the grotesque cause of the outbreak, which was due to involuntary cannibalism among cattle. In order to promote their growth, the animals were fed protein supplements that included brain and spinal cord tissue from other cattle. Prion diseases can extremely rarely occur spontaneously in animals, or due to rare genetic defects; when the remains of these animals are mixed into the food of hundreds of other animals, catastrophe results. A similar but even more macabre epidemic of prion disease, involving human rather than bovine cannibalism, spread through the Fore people of Papua New Guinea starting in the early 20th century, in the wake of their adopting 'mortuary cannibalism'—the practice of ceremonially eating their dead relatives—and vanished again after the abandonment of cannibalism in the mid-20th century.

What is the outlook for the control of infectious diseases over the next few decades? What are the likely impacts of infectious disease on your health and welfare, or on your family's, from diseases that are already present, or from newly emerging ones? How will the ecology and evolution of disease change in the future?

The first thing we know is that 'plus ça change, plus c'est la même chose' (the more things change, the more they stay the same). Our understanding of how diseases are transmitted, and the development of vaccines and treatments that can close the compatibility filter, has revolutionized disease management, but the basic processes driving the disease ecosystem remain the same. Humans have had some resounding successes: we have completely eradicated smallpox and rinderpest, and we can realistically consider the possibility of polio and measles eradication even though the last steps are proving to be immensely difficult for social, political, and economic reasons. Even though it is hard to imagine eradicating HIV, we have developed treatments that allow infected people (at least those with access to good medical care) to tolerate the disease and live out their regular lifespan.

However, we have also lost ground. Tuberculosis has re-emerged, especially in conjunction with HIV; the first optimistic decades of malaria control ended in retreat; and new diseases such as Lyme disease, West Nile virus, and H1N1 influenza have continued to spill over from animal populations. Perhaps the scariest failures have been our glimpses of the potential of drug and antibiotic resistance in MRSA or malaria or multiply resistant tuberculosis, where we are once again forced to contemplate the spectre of untreatable diseases.

A future free of infectious disease is simply unrealistic. Living things have parasitized one another since the beginning of life itself, and no amount of intervention will alter that. New diseases will be created by mutation or recombination of existing ones and by spillover from animal populations, and existing diseases will continually evolve to escape our methods of control. What is attainable, however, is minimizing the impact of disease while understanding that it will always be with us. We *can* slow or stop pandemics, and we *can* reduce the amount of death and misery that diseases cause, even if we can never fully conquer them.

What has changed in our understanding of infectious diseases over the last fifty years? During that period, we moved from population-level treatment to individual treatment. What we have learned in this progression is that population-level treatment, in contrast to curing individuals after they have already been infected, is still invaluable in stopping disease. The simplest way to minimize the impact of disease is to minimize its incidence in the first place. We are learning that there is synergy between population-level and individual-level approaches to prevent disease. The phenomenon of herd immunity is one such example (see Chapter 2).

As our case studies have illustrated, the organisms that cause disease evolve. Tuberculosis is re-emerging in part because the bacteria that cause it have evolved antibiotic resistance. HIV evolved to survive better in humans following its host shift from other primates. But remember—mutations happen at random. So too do encounters between relatively harmless bacteria with bacteria or viruses carrying dangerous pathogenicity genes. Because of that inherent randomness, the fewer organisms that are present, the less likely it is that they will evolve to become more virulent. Think of it this way: if there are twenty viruses, and a mutation that makes them resistant to an antiviral agent happens only one in a million times, it's quite improbable that one of them will experience that rare mutation. But if there are a billion of them, the event is practically inevitable. So by keeping the numbers of organisms that infect us low through population-level interventions like effective vaccination or quarantine, we reduce the probability that they will evolve to become more dangerous. Again, an ounce of prevention is worth a pound of cure.

One of the lessons from past failures of disease control is that the miracles of modern molecular biology have limitations. Vaccines are simplest to develop when the human body already has a quick and effective immune response. For diseases like HIV, malaria, or tuberculosis that use evolutionary tricks such as costume-switching to evade the immune response, we may never be able to achieve the same cheap, effective vaccines that eradicated smallpox and have brought measles and polio to the brink of eradication.

Even as we have learned the limitations of magic bullets, we have new technological applications that can help with both detection of disease organisms and with healing. Identification of viruses or testing bacteria for antibiotic resistance used to take days or weeks. For example, virus classification involved careful microscopic inspection or time-consuming immunological techniques. Testing for resistance involved assessing the ability of bacteria to grow on plates containing various antibiotics. Now we can diagnose and characterize bacteria and viruses by sequencing their genomes within hours. Moreover, these techniques are no longer relegated to skilled technicians in laboratories; sequencing technologies suitable for unprocessed samples (such as saliva or blood) under field conditions are now available, and costs are dropping by the month. Such genotyping technologies may also be useful in bacterial infections, for tailoring the correct sort of phage to use against them as part of phage therapy.

Another lesson we have learned is the power, as well as the limitations, of changing human behaviour. We can easily close the encounter filter for many diseases by checking thoroughly for ticks after we go into the woods, stopping the exchange of bodily fluids with strangers, and staying home (or keeping our kids home) when we develop a cough. However, the practical and economic costs of changing our behaviour often mean that we keep exposing ourselves, and others, even when the solutions seem (on the surface) to be relatively simple and even when the consequences (such as contracting HIV) are dire. For you, the reader of this book, this is relatively good news; there are lots of simple ways that you can prevent your own infection, or, if you are infected, stop transmitting disease to others. But humans as a whole are stubborn creatures, and we have many conflicting priorities—earning a living or simply saving a little bit of time may often trump the practices that could save us, or others, from infection.

One of the important frontiers in disease control is figuring out better ways to honestly but effectively inform the public about the dangers of disease and the methods that are in their hands for controlling it. Sometimes the interests of the individual and the population diverge. For example, staying home from work when we're sick might be a bad individual decision on purely selfish grounds, because it costs us a day's pay or a boss's goodwill, even if it benefits our co-workers. We must do a better job at designing policies that encourage compliance with public health goals, using a sensible combination of carrots and sticks without unduly restricting individual freedoms.

The continuing pressure of humanity on the environment is another thing that has changed, but has also stayed the same. Urbanization and increased population growth increase the rates at which humans contract new pathogens, largely carried by animals. As we move into previously uncolonized habitats, or as we modify our environments, encounter rates with animals and the parasites they carry increase. This does not just apply to tropical diseases, but also to temperate diseases (recall Lyme disease). Humans are changing their environment in huge numbers of ways—cleaning our water, aggregating in modern mega-cities, clearing tropical forest—that will change our epidemiological landscapes both for better and for worse.

Epidemiologists are locked in an intense debate over the possible effects of the largest-scale uncontrolled experiment in history—the release of CO_2 from fossil fuels into the atmosphere, and the concomitant changes in global climate—on disease prevalence. On the one hand, there is no question that ecological change brings about epidemiological change; many species' ranges have already been observed to shift in response to climate change, and it makes sense that this would apply to insect vectors such as mosquitoes as well. In particular locations, such as the highlands of East Africa, increasing temperatures do indeed seem to have driven increases in the incidence of malaria. But the regional effects of climate change are complex, involving changes in variability, seasonal patterns and the hydrological cycle as well as the overall temperature. Add that to the complexity and unpredictability of interactions of ecological systems with regional climate, and other scientists say that although we can say with certainty that climate change will have *some* effect on disease, it is hard to know exactly what it will be.

Mosquitoes are an interesting problem. At first glance, getting rid of mosquitoes, at least the ones that we know vector particularly devastating diseases, seems like a good idea. Indeed, it has recently been argued that scientists have become too narrowly focused on problems of drug resistance of malaria, and that we could ignore that altogether if we decided to launch an attack on mosquitoes. Eliminating mosquitoes, however, requires interventions like draining wetlands and/or use of pesticides that devastate many other species. And, of course, mosquitoes become resistant to insecticides, even as malaria becomes resistant to antimalarial drugs. However, there's a larger point to be made here: we mustn't allow our thinking about infectious disease to stagnate. Overconfidence in any one solution (antimalarial drugs), or overfocus on any part of the multifaceted problem that is infectious disease (for example, solely on parasite resistance), limits our ability to solve any kind of problem.

Human health is not just about vanquishing wicked parasites, either with magic bullets, everyday practice, or even both. The parasites are embedded in the same natural system that we are. Though we have spent little time discussing it in this book, human sociology also has huge effects on the spread of infectious disease. In the New Testament, the Four Horsemen of the Apocalypse are War, Famine, Pestilence, and Death. There's a reason they are grouped together: perhaps the most effective way to rid ourselves of the worst of infectious disease would be to achieve world peace and global prosperity. Sadly, a broader understanding of ecology and evolution as they pertain to infectious disease seems rather more attainable.

Plus ça change, plus c'est la même chose. As we write, an outbreak of the Ebola virus has already killed thousands of people in western Africa. The emergence of Ebola underscores many of the points we have made throughout this book. Ebola is another example of a zoonotic disease. The virus likely came to us from bats, and while the shift from bats to people is uncommon, genetic analysis of a variety of strains tells us that it has happened several times. A technical fix to close the compatibility filter is not possible in the short term—as yet, we have no reliable vaccine or drug treatment for Ebola—but hydration and other support does seem to improve outcomes. Quarantines could be effective to close the encounter filter, but would have been most effective in the early stages of the epidemic. The local postcolonial infrastructure could not, and cannot, deal with the challenges of Ebola alone, and the attention of the world was elsewhere. This changed abruptly when, as with almost every other disease we have discussed, global travel enabled the spread of Ebola to North America and Europe. Thus far, transmission outside of Africa has been stopped promptly.

As with HIV, fear of Ebola has stigmatized the disease. People are understandably attempting to hide infection in themselves or their families, further complicating attempts to understand the scope and dynamics of the epidemic. There has been much discussion of the importance of not stigmatizing international healthcare workers returning to their homes following service in Africa, while dealing sensibly with the risk and fear of contagion among their compatriots. Fear has also led to food scarcity in the areas of sub-Saharan Africa where the epidemic is the worst, making quarantines even more challenging, and creating an additional crisis.

Ebola terrifies people in part because of the mode of transmission, and in part because the fatality rate, particularly in Africa, is high. All the bodily fluids of a person with an active Ebola infection—particularly anyone who has died from the disease—are loaded with infectious virus. However, Ebola's grisly mode of transmission means that the encounter filter is relatively small. You only need to come in contact with a few virus particles to get sick. But with the small encounter filter, people other than healthcare workers and those who take care of the dead are unlikely to become sick, because it is unlikely that they will come into contact with contaminated bodily fluids. (Unfortunately, traditional African customs often mean that many of a dead person's relatives come in contact with the body before and during the funeral.) For example, family members of Thomas Duncan, the first person to be diagnosed with Ebola in the US who subsequently died from the disease, did not become sick despite living with him for several days after he became contagious. Two of the nurses caring for Duncan in a hospital did become infected, but happily they recovered.

At the time of writing it is difficult to predict the trajectory of the Ebola epidemic. However, by the time this book is in the hands of a reader, it seems virtually inevitable that yet another infectious disease will be emerging. Plus ça change... Apologize politely to the masked stranger who comes to your party uninvited, and explain that s/he will have to indulge you in hand washing before visiting the buffet; regale your guests with True Stories of effective vaccination campaigns; and take any medications you are given as directed (but feel free to discuss them with your doctor!). We cannot hope to live in a world free of infectious disease, but if we act wisely, we can live more safely.

Further reading

Chapter 1: Introduction

Blake, John B. 1952. 'The Inoculation Controversy in Boston: 1721–1722'. *The New England Quarterly* 25 (4): 489–506.

Brault, Aaron C., Claire Y.-H. Huang, Stanley A. Langevin, Richard M. Kinney, Richard A. Bowen, Wanichaya N. Ramey, Nicholas A. Panella, Edward C. Holmes, Ann M. Powers, and Barry R. Miller. 2007. 'A Single Positively Selected West Nile Viral Mutation Confers Increased Virogenesis in American Crows'. *Nature Genetics* 39 (9): 1162–6.

Combes, Claude. 2005. *The Art of Being a Parasite*. Chicago, IL: University of Chicago Press.

Davies, Julian. 1995. 'Vicious Circles: Looking Back on Resistance Plasmids'. *Genetics* 139 (4): 1465.

D'Costa, Vanessa M., Christine E. King, Lindsay Kalan, Mariya Morar, Wilson W. L. Sung, Carsten Schwarz, Duane Froese, et al. 2011. 'Antibiotic Resistance Is Ancient'. *Nature* 477 (7365): 457–61.

Garrett, Laurie. 1995. *The Coming Plague: Newly Emerging Diseases in a World Out of Balance*. Reprint edition. New York: Penguin Books.

Mackowiak, Philip A., and Paul S. Sehdev. 2002. 'The Origin of Quarantine'. *Clinical Infectious Diseases* 35 (9): 1071–2.

Miranda, Mary Elizabeth G., and Noel Lee J. Miranda. 2011. 'Reston Ebolavirus in Humans and Animals in the Philippines: A Review'. *Journal of Infectious Diseases* 204 (suppl. 3): S757–60.

Stearns, Stephen C., and Jacob C. Koella. 2008. *Evolution in Health and Disease*. 2nd edition. Oxford; New York: Oxford University Press.

Chapter 2: Transmission at different scales

Bernoulli, Daniel, and Sally Blower. 2004. 'An Attempt at a New Analysis of the Mortality Caused by Smallpox and of the Advantages of Inoculation to Prevent It'. *Reviews in Medical Virology* 14 (5): 275–88.

Combes, Claude. 2004. *Parasitism: The Ecology and Evolution of Intimate Interactions*. Translated by Isaure de Buron and Vincent A. Connors. Chicago: University Of Chicago Press.

Hethcote, Herbert W. 1994. 'A Thousand and One Epidemic Models'. In *Frontiers in Mathematical Biology*, edited by Simon A. Levin, 504–15. Lecture Notes in Biomathematics 100. Berlin: Springer.

Keeling, Matthew James, and Pejman Rohani. 2008. *Modeling Infectious Diseases in Humans and Animals*. Princeton: Princeton University Press.

McGovern, B., E. Doyle, L. E. Fenelon, and S. F. FitzGerald. 2010. 'The Necktie As a Potential Vector of Infection: Are Doctors Happy to Do Without?' *The Journal of Hospital Infection* 75 (2): 138–9.

Thomas, Y., G. Vogel, W. Wunderli, P. Suter, M. Witschi, D. Koch, C. Tapparel, and L. Kaiser. 2008. 'Survival of Influenza Virus on Banknotes'. *Applied and Environmental Microbiology* 74 (10): 3002–7.

Chapter 3: Influenza

Adams, Patrick. 2012. 'The Influenza Enigma'. *Bulletin of the World Health Organization* 90 (4): 245.

Cohen, Jon, and David Malakoff. 2012. 'On Second Thought, Flu Papers Get Go-Ahead'. *Science* 336 (6077): 19–20.

Dushoff, Jonathan, Joshua B. Plotkin, Cécile Viboud, David J. D. Earn, and Lone Simonsen. 2006. 'Mortality Due to Influenza in the United States: An Annualized Regression Approach Using Multiple-Cause Mortality Data'. *American Journal of Epidemiology* 163 (2): 181–7.

Lipsitch, M., and C. Viboud. 2009. 'Influenza Seasonality: Lifting the Fog'. *Proceedings of the National Academy of Sciences* 106 (10): 3645–6.

Loeb, M., M.L. Russell, L. Moss, et al. 2010. 'Effect of Influenza Vaccination of Children on Infection Rates in Hutterite Communities: A Randomized Trial'. *JAMA* 303 (10): 943–50.

Mereckiene, Jolita, Suzanne Cotter, F. D'Ancona, C. Giambi, A. Nicoll, Daniel Levy-Bruhl, P. L. Lopalco, et al. 2010. 'Differences in National Influenza Vaccination Policies Across the European Union, Norway and Iceland 2008–2009'. <https://lenus.ie/hse/handle/10147/125883>.
Nobusawa, Eri, and Katsuhiko Sato. 2006. 'Comparison of the Mutation Rates of Human Influenza A and B Viruses'. *Journal of Virology* 80 (7): 3675–8.
Roach, Jared C., Gustavo Glusman, Arian F. A. Smit, Chad D. Huff, Robert Hubley, Paul T. Shannon, Lee Rowen, et al. 2010. 'Analysis of Genetic Inheritance in a Family Quartet by Whole-Genome Sequencing'. *Science* 328 (5978): 636–9.
Schuchat, Anne. 2010. 'CDC Response: H1N1 Presentation for Immunization Update 2010'. Centers for Disease Control and Prevention, 27 July. <http://www.cdc.gov/h1n1flu/imm_update_transcript.htm>.
Simonsen, Lone, Peter Spreeuwenberg, Roger Lustig, Robert J. Taylor, Douglas M. Fleming, Madelon Kroneman, Maria D. Van Kerkhove, Anthony W. Mounts, W. John Paget, and the GLaMOR Collaborating Teams. 2013. 'Global Mortality Estimates for the 2009 Influenza Pandemic from the GLaMOR Project: A Modeling Study'. *PLoS Med* 10 (11): e1001558.
Tamerius, James, Martha I. Nelson, Steven Z. Zhou, Cécile Viboud, Mark A. Miller, and Wladimir J. Alonso. 2011. 'Global Influenza Seasonality: Reconciling Patterns across Temperate and Tropical Regions'. *Environmental Health Perspectives* 119 (4): 439–45.

Chapter 4: HIV

Faria, Nuno R., Andrew Rambaut, Marc A. Suchard, Guy Baele, Trevor Bedford, Melissa J. Ward, Andrew J. Tatem, et al. 2014. 'The Early Spread and Epidemic Ignition of HIV-1 in Human Populations'. *Science* 346 (6205): 56–61.
Frank, Steven A. 2002. *Immunology and Evolution of Infectious Disease*. Princeton, NJ: Princeton University Press.
Fraser, C., K. Lythgoe, G. E. Leventhal, G. Shirreff, T. D. Hollingsworth, S. Alizon, and S. Bonhoeffer. 2014. 'Virulence and Pathogenesis of HIV-1 Infection: An Evolutionary Perspective'. *Science* 343 (6177).
Holmes, Edward C. 2009. *The Evolution and Emergence of RNA Viruses*. Oxford: Oxford University Press.

Marx, Preston A., Phillip G. Alcabes, and Ernest Drucker. 2001. 'Serial Human Passage of Simian Immunodeficiency Virus by Unsterile Injections and the Emergence of Epidemic Human Immunodeficiency Virus in Africa'. *Philosophical Transactions of the Royal Society B: Biological Sciences* 356 (1410): 911–20.

Mild, Mattias, Rebecca R. Gray, Anders Kvist, Philippe Lemey, Maureen M. Goodenow, Eva Maria Fenyö, Jan Albert, Marco Salemi, Joakim Esbjörnsson, and Patrik Medstrand. 2013. 'High Intrapatient HIV-1 Evolutionary Rate Is Associated with CCR5-to-CXCR4 Coreceptor Switch'. *Infection, Genetics and Evolution* 19 (October): 369–77.

Müller, Viktor, and Sebastian Bonhoeffer. 2008. 'Intra-Host Dynamics and Evolution of HIV Infection'. In *Origin and Evolution of Viruses*, 2nd edition, edited by Esteban Domingo, Colin R. Parrish, and John J. Holland, 279–301. London: Academic Press.

Novembre, John, and Eunjung Han. 2012. 'Human Population Structure and the Adaptive Response to Pathogen-Induced Selection Pressures'. *Philosophical Transactions of the Royal Society B: Biological Sciences* 367 (1590): 878–86.

Sharp, Paul M., and Beatrice H. Hahn. 2011. 'Origins of HIV and the AIDS Pandemic'. *Cold Spring Harbor Perspectives in Medicine* 1 (1): a006841.

Chapter 5: Cholera

Colwell, Rita R. 1996. 'Global Climate and Infectious Disease: The Cholera Paradigm'. *Science*, New Series, 274 (5295): 2025–31.

Jubair, Mohamma, J. Glenn Morris, and Afsar Ali. 2012. 'Survival of *Vibrio cholerae* in Nutrient-Poor Environments Is Associated with a Novel "Persister" Phenotype'. *PLoS ONE* 7 (9): e45187.

Kaper, J. B., J. G. Morris, and M. M. Levine. 1995. 'Cholera'. *Clinical Microbiology Reviews* 8 (1): 48–86.

Kitaoka, Maya, Sarah T. Miyata, Daniel Unterweger, and Stefan Pukatzki. 2011. 'Antibiotic Resistance Mechanisms of *Vibrio cholerae*'. *Journal of Medical Microbiology* 60 (4): 397–407.

Morris, J. Glenn. 2011. 'Cholera: Modern Pandemic Disease of Ancient Lineage'. *Emerging Infectious Diseases* 17 (11).

Nelson, Eric J., Ashrafuzzaman Chowdhury, James Flynn, Stefan Schild, Lori Bourassa, Yue Shao, Regina C. LaRocque, Stephen B. Calderwood, Firdausi Qadri, and Andrew Camilli. 2008.

'Transmission of *Vibrio cholerae* Is Antagonized by Lytic Phage and Entry into the Aquatic Environment'. *PLoS Pathog* 4 (10): e1000187.

Zuger, Abigail. 2011. 'Small Fixes: Folding Saris to Filter Cholera-Contaminated Water'. *The New York Times*, 26 September. <http://www.nytimes.com/2011/09/27/health/27sari.html>.

Chapter 6: Malaria

Faust, E. C. 1951. 'The History of Malaria in the United States'. *American Scientist* 39 (1): 121–30.

Gladwell, Malcolm. 2001. 'The Mosquito Killer'. *The New Yorker*, 2 July. <http://www.newyorker.com/magazine/2001/07/02/the-mosquito-killer>.

Hedrick, Philip W. 2012. 'Resistance to Malaria in Humans: The Impact of Strong, Recent Selection'. *Malaria Journal* 11 (October): 349.

Kantele, Anu, and T. Sakari Jokiranta. 2011. 'Review of Cases with the Emerging Fifth Human Malaria Parasite, *Plasmodium knowlesi*'. *Clinical Infectious Diseases* 52 (11): 1356–62.

Klayman, D. L. 1985. 'Qinghaosu (artemisinin): An Antimalarial Drug from China'. *Science* 228 (4703): 1049–55.

Krief, Sabrina, Ananias A. Escalante, M. Andreina Pacheco, Lawrence Mugisha, Claudine André, Michel Halbwax, Anne Fischer, et al. 2010. 'On the Diversity of Malaria Parasites in African Apes and the Origin of *Plasmodium falciparum* from Bonobos'. *PLoS Pathog* 6 (2): e1000765.

Lalremruata, Albert, Markus Ball, Raffaella Bianucci, Beatrix Welte, Andreas G. Nerlich, Jürgen F. J. Kun, and Carsten M. Pusch. 2013. 'Molecular Identification of Falciparum Malaria and Human Tuberculosis Co-Infections in Mummies from the Fayum Depression (Lower Egypt)'. *PLoS ONE* 8 (4): e60307.

Liu, Weimin, Yingying Li, Gerald H. Learn, Rebecca S. Rudicell, Joel D. Robertson, Brandon F. Keele, Jean-Bosco N. Ndjango, et al. 2010a. 'Origin of the Human Malaria Parasite *Plasmodium falciparum* in Gorillas'. *Nature* 467 (7314): 420–5.

Liu, Weimin, Yingying Li, Katharina S. Shaw, Gerald H. Learn, Lindsey J. Plenderleith, Jordan A. Malenke, Sesh A. Sundararaman, et al. 2014. 'African Origin of the Malaria Parasite *Plasmodium vivax*'. *Nature Communications* 5 (February).

Nosten, François H. 2014. 'How to Beat Malaria, Once and for All'. *The New York Times*, 7 June. <http://www.nytimes.com/2014/06/08/opinion/sunday/how-to-beat-malaria-once-and-for-all.html>.

Outlaw, Diana C., and Robert E. Ricklefs. 2011. 'Rerooting the Evolutionary Tree of Malaria Parasites'. *Proceedings of the National Academy of Sciences* 108 (32): 13183–7.

Piel, Frédéric B., Anand P. Patil, Rosalind E. Howes, Oscar A. Nyangiri, Peter W. Gething, Thomas N. Williams, David J. Weatherall, and Simon I. Hay. 2010. 'Global Distribution of the Sickle Cell Gene and Geographical Confirmation of the Malaria Hypothesis'. *Nature Communications* 1: 104.

Poinar, G., and S. R. Telford. 2005. '*Paleohaemoproteus burmacis* Gen. N., Sp. N. (Haemospororida: Plasmodiidae) from an Early Cretaceous Biting Midge (Diptera: Ceratopogonidae)'. *Parasitology* 131 (01): 79–84.

Rich, Stephen M., Monica C. Licht, Richard R. Hudson, and Francisco J. Ayala. 1998. 'Malaria's Eve: Evidence of a Recent Population Bottleneck throughout the World Populations of *Plasmodium falciparum*'. *Proceedings of the National Academy of Sciences* 95 (8): 4425–30.

Rich, Stephen M., and Guang Xu. 2011. 'Resolving the Phylogeny of Malaria Parasites'. *Proceedings of the National Academy of Sciences* 108 (32): 12973–4.

Tishkoff, Sarah A., Robert Varkonyi, Nelie Cahinhinan, Salem Abbes, George Argyropoulos, Giovanni Destro-Bisol, Anthi Drousiotou, et al. 2001. 'Haplotype Diversity and Linkage Disequilibrium at Human G6PD: Recent Origin of Alleles that Confer Malarial Resistance'. *Science* 293 (5529): 455–62.

Webb, James L. A. 2009. 'The Long Shadow of Malaria Interventions in Tropical Africa'. *The Lancet* 374 (9705): 1883–4.

Chapter 7: *Batrachochytrium dendrobatidis*

Blaustein, Andrew R., John M. Romansic, Erin A. Scheessele, Barbara A. Han, Allan P. Pessier, and Joyce E. Longcore. 2005. 'Interspecific Variation in Susceptibility of Frog Tadpoles to the Pathogenic Fungus *Batrachochytrium dendrobatidis*. *Conservation Biology* 19 (5): 1460–8.

Briggs, Cheryl J., Vance T. Vredenburg, Roland A. Knapp, and Lara J. Rachowicz. 2005. 'Investigating the Population-Level Effects of

Chytridiomycosis: An Emerging Infectious Disease of Amphibians'. *Ecology* 86 (12): 3149–59.
Burke, Katie L. 2013. 'Probiotics for Frogs'. *American Scientist* 100 (3): 190.
Fisher, Matthew C., Trenton W. J. Garner, and Susan F. Walker. 2009. 'Global Emergence of *Batrachochytrium dendrobatidis* and Amphibian Chytridiomycosis in Space, Time, and Host'. *Annual Review of Microbiology* 63 (1): 291–310.
Gervasi, Stephanie S., Jenny Urbina, Jessica Hua, Tara Chestnut, Rick A. Relyea, and Andrew R. Blaustein. 2013. 'Experimental Evidence for American Bullfrog (*Lithobates catesbeianus*) Susceptibility to Chytrid Fungus (*Batrachochytrium dendrobatidis*)'. *EcoHealth* 10 (2): 166–71.
Kilpatrick, A. Marm, Cheryl J. Briggs, and Peter Daszak. 2010. 'The Ecology and Impact of Chytridiomycosis: An Emerging Disease of Amphibians'. *Trends in Ecology & Evolution* 25 (2): 109–18.
Lips, Karen R., Jay Diffendorfer, Joseph R. Mendelson III, and Michael W. Sears. 2008. 'Riding the Wave: Reconciling the Roles of Disease and Climate Change in Amphibian Declines'. *PLoS Biol* 6 (3): e72.
Martel, An, Annemarieke Spitzen-van der Sluijs, Mark Blooi, Wim Bert, Richard Ducatelle, Matthew C. Fisher, Antonius Woeltjes, et al. 2013. '*Batrachochytrium salamandrivorans* Sp. Nov. Causes Lethal Chytridiomycosis in Amphibians'. *Proceedings of the National Academy of Sciences* 110 (38): 15325–9.
McMahon, Taegan A., Laura A. Brannelly, Matthew W. H. Chatfield, Pieter T. J. Johnson, Maxwell B. Joseph, Valerie J. McKenzie, Corinne L. Richards-Zawacki, Matthew D. Venesky, and Jason R. Rohr. 2013. 'Chytrid Fungus *Batrachochytrium dendrobatidis* Has Nonamphibian Hosts and Releases Chemicals that Cause Pathology in the Absence of Infection'. *Proceedings of the National Academy of Sciences* 110 (1): 210–15.
McMahon, Taegan A., Brittany F. Sears, Matthew D. Venesky, Scott M. Bessler, Jenise M. Brown, Kaitlin Deutsch, Neal T. Halstead, et al. 2014. 'Amphibians Acquire Resistance to Live and Dead Fungus Overcoming Fungal Immunosuppression'. *Nature* 511 (7508): 224–7.
Rachowicz, Lara J., Roland A. Knapp, Jess A. T. Morgan, Mary J. Stice, Vance T. Vredenburg, John M. Parker, and Cheryl J. Briggs. 2006. 'Emerging Infectious Disease As a Proximate Cause of Amphibian Mass Mortality'. *Ecology* 87 (7): 1671–83.

Rodriguez, D., C. G. Becker, N. C. Pupin, C. F. B. Haddad, and K. R. Zamudio. 2014. 'Long-Term Endemism of Two Highly Divergent Lineages of the Amphibian-Killing Fungus in the Atlantic Forest of Brazil'. *Molecular Ecology* 23 (4): 774–87.

Rosenblum, Erica Bree, Timothy Y. James, Kelly R. Zamudio, Thomas J. Poorten, Dan Ilut, David Rodriguez, Jonathan M. Eastman, et al. 2013. 'Complex History of the Amphibian-Killing Chytrid Fungus Revealed with Genome Resequencing Data'. *Proceedings of the National Academy of Sciences* 110 (23): 9385–90.

Rohr, Jason R., and Thomas R. Raffel. 2010. 'Linking Global Climate and Temperature Variability to Widespread Amphibian Declines Putatively Caused by Disease'. *Proceedings of the National Academy of Sciences* 107 (18): 8269–74.

Chapter 8: Looking ahead

Brown, P., R. G. Will, R. Bradley, D. M. Asher, and L. Detwiler. 2001. 'Bovine Spongiform Encephalopathy and Variant Creutzfeldt-Jakob Disease: Background, Evolution, and Current Concerns'. *Emerging Infectious Diseases* 7 (1): 6–16.

Fisman, David, Edwin Khoo, and Ashleigh Tuite. 2014. 'Early Epidemic Dynamics of the West African 2014 Ebola Outbreak: Estimates Derived with a Simple Two-Parameter Model'. *PLOS Currents Outbreaks*. 8 September. Edition 1.

Hewlett, Barry, and Bonnie Hewlett. 2007. *Ebola, Culture and Politics: The Anthropology of an Emerging Disease*. Andover: Cengage Learning.

Reiter, Paul, Christopher J. Thomas, Peter M. Atkinson, Simon I. Hay, Sarah E. Randolph, David J. Rogers, G. Dennis Shanks, Robert W. Snow, and Andrew Spielman. 2004. 'Global Warming and Malaria: A Call for Accuracy'. *The Lancet Infectious Diseases* 4 (6): 323–4.

Suzuki, Y., and T. Gojobori. 1997. 'The Origin and Evolution of Ebola and Marburg Viruses'. *Molecular Biology and Evolution* 14 (8): 800–6.

“牛津通识读本”已出书目

古典哲学的趣味
人生的意义
文学理论入门
大众经济学
历史之源
设计，无处不在
生活中的心理学
政治的历史与边界
哲学的思与惑
资本主义
美国总统制
海德格尔
我们时代的伦理学
卡夫卡是谁
考古学的过去与未来
天文学简史
社会学的意识
康德
尼采
亚里士多德的世界
西方艺术新论
全球化面面观
简明逻辑学
法哲学：价值与事实
政治哲学与幸福根基
选择理论
后殖民主义与世界格局
福柯
缤纷的语言学
达达和超现实主义
佛学概论
维特根斯坦与哲学
科学哲学
印度哲学祛魅
克尔凯郭尔
科学革命
广告
数学
叔本华
笛卡尔
基督教神学
犹太人与犹太教
现代日本
罗兰·巴特
马基雅维里
全球经济史
进化
性存在
量子理论
牛顿新传
国际移民
哈贝马斯
医学伦理
黑格尔
地球
记忆
法律
中国文学
托克维尔
休谟
分子
法国大革命
丝绸之路
民族主义
科幻作品
罗素
美国政党与选举
美国最高法院
纪录片
大萧条与罗斯福新政
领导力
无神论
罗马共和国
美国国会
民主
英格兰文学
现代主义
网络
自闭症
德里达
浪漫主义

批判理论
电影
俄罗斯文学
古典文学
大数据
洛克
幸福
免疫系统
银行学

德国文学
戏剧
腐败
医事法
癌症
植物
法语文学
微观经济学

儿童心理学
时装
现代拉丁美洲文学
卢梭
隐私
电影音乐
抑郁症
传染病